Key Skills for Housing Adaptations

The Essential Guide for Newly Qualified Occupational Therapists
Transition to Practice
Edited by Ruth Parker and Julia Badger
ISBN 978 1 78592 268 8
eISBN 978 1 78450 558 5

of related interest

Antiracist Occupational Therapy
Unsettling the Status Quo
Edited by Musharrat J. Ahmed-Landeryou
Foreword by Professor Elelwani Ramugondo
ISBN 978 1 83997 574 5
eISBN 978 1 83997 575 2

The Core Concepts of Occupational Therapy
A Dynamic Framework for Practice
Jennifer Creek
ISBN 978 1 84905 007 4
eISBN 978 0 85700 362 1

Mindfulness-Based Therapy for Managing Fatigue
Supporting People with ME/CFS, Fibromyalgia and Long Covid
Fiona McKechnie
Forewords by Rebecca Crane and Dh Taravajra
ISBN 978 1 83997 345 1
eISBN 978 1 83997 346 8

KEY SKILLS FOR HOUSING ADAPTATIONS

A Workbook for Occupational Therapists and Students

RUTH PARKER AND **DAVID OWEN**
WITH **JULIA BADGER**

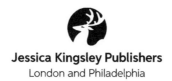

Jessica Kingsley Publishers
London and Philadelphia

First published in Great Britain in 2024 by Jessica Kingsley Publishers
An imprint of John Murray Press

1

A CIP catalogue record for this title is available from the
British Library and the Library of Congress

ISBN 978 1 83997 446 5
eISBN 978 1 83997 447 2

Printed and bound in Great Britain by CPI Group

Jessica Kingsley Publishers' policy is to use papers that are natural, renewable and recyclable
products and made from wood grown in sustainable forests. The logging and manufacturing
processes are expected to conform to the environmental regulations of the country of origin.

Jessica Kingsley Publishers
Carmelite House
50 Victoria Embankment
London EC4Y 0DZ

www.jkp.com

John Murray Press
Part of Hodder & Stoughton Ltd
An Hachette Company

Contents

Contributors

Ruth Parker has worked as an occupational therapist in social care since 2001, moving to the Children with Disabilities team in 2005. Reflecting her interest in the built environment and adaptations she completed an MSc in Accessibility and Inclusive Design, which led to a PhD investigating the impact of choice and compromise on the design of children's play parks. She has completed research with Elizabeth Cooper on the long-term effectiveness of recommendations for adaptations made by occupational therapists in Lincolnshire, and co-edited *The Essential Guide for Newly Qualified Occupational Therapists* with Julia Badger.

David Owen is the current Chair of the Royal College of Occupational Therapists Specialist Section – Housing, holding this position since summer 2021. David has a background working in adult social care, and in the past six years specializing in housing. David has lectured at the University of South Wales on the Occupational Therapy degree and is now a senior practitioner in housing for South Gloucestershire Council.

Julia Badger has worked across a number of sectors since graduating as an occupational therapist, with experience in adult and children's social care, the NHS and an integrated community equipment service. Julia is currently working in the NHS on a specialist stroke unit. With Ruth Parker, Julia co-edited *The Essential Guide for Newly Qualified Occupational Therapists*.

Elizabeth Cooper graduated from the Derby Occupational Therapy School in 1973, and then spent 37 years in a variety of roles within the NHS. In 2015 Elizabeth joined Lincolnshire County Council as Practice Lead for Adult Social Care Occupational Therapy, which included the organization of two conferences and research with Ruth Parker investigating the long-term effectiveness of recommendations for adaptations made by occupational therapists in Lincolnshire. Elizabeth co-created and taught an 'Introduction to Adaptions' course for those new to this area of practice. Elizabeth recently retired from practice, but retains an active interest in occupational therapy.

Andrea Cox is an experienced building surveyor working for North Kesteven District Council with a remit to promote independence through the design of housing adaptations, taking into consideration families' and clients' disability needs within the scope of the built environment. Andrea has contributed images and architectural drawings to illustrate information and for use with the case studies.

Shane Elliott works as Housing and Health Lead in a post that is joint-funded by the Department of Health and the Northern Ireland Housing Executive. The role seeks to ensure that health and housing staff work collaboratively to provide the best and most appropriate housing solution for people with disabilities. He provides specialist advice, training and expertise to a range of staff, and supports the Chief Allied Health Professions Officer in responding to Northern Ireland Executive business, ministerial briefs and Assembly questions.

Sarah Harris graduated from the University of Salford in 2008. She currently works as Assessment Team Manager for Manchester City Council, and has worked for the Council for over 30 years. Most of her experience has been in equipment and adaptations, which has involved assessing children and adults with complex needs for equipment, and minor and major adaptations. During this time she has also been involved in the design consultation of many extra-care schemes in Manchester and the award-winning BBC *DIY SOS Big Build* veterans village. She also worked for the adapted homes team at Manchester Move rehousing service for five years, reletting adapted properties and awarding medical priority to rehousing applications. Sarah was the northwest representative for the Royal College of Occupational Therapists Specialist Section (Housing) between 2011 and 2019.

Ammelia May is an occupational therapist with experience working with children with disabilities in Children's Services including assessment and recommendation for complex housing adaptations. After working with Children's Services she moved to a clinical role in the NHS. Ammelia is currently Clinical Lead Occupational Therapist at Hollybank Trust, a charity supporting people with profound and multiple learning disabilities.

Jill Pritchard is an occupational therapist specializing in housing issues, and is also a workplace change consultant. Working as an independent practitioner she has 30 years' experience in social care and housing. Jill works with the Scottish Government's Joint Improvement Team, and supports health, housing and social care partnerships via the ihub within Healthcare Improvement Scotland. Jill also works to improve the delivery of adaptations, housing solutions and place-based interventions at operational and strategic levels across a number of sectors promoting occupational therapy and staffing resources to produce better outcomes for people. She co-authored the *Inclusive Living Toolkit*, and is passionate about mainstreaming inclusive design and inclusive living. She is the Scotland representative for RCOT Specialist Section – Housing and Vice Chair of Horizon Housing Association.

Kate Sheehan is an occupational therapist with 36 years of clinical experience, having graduated from the Derby Occupational Therapy School in 1987. Kate is one of the Directors of The OT Service, which provides consultancy as well as occupational therapy to individuals, case managers and solicitors. Her specialist area of practice is accessible housing design, championing the need to understand the meaning of 'home' to an individual, and how poorly designed modifications can have a significant impact on wellbeing. Kate is working with the Department for Levelling Up, Housing and Communities on the development of an accessible built environment, and co-authored the *Wheelchair Housing Design Guide* for the Centre for Accessible Environments. Kate was involved in the newly funded research project into wheelchair space standards to inform the revised Part M of the Building Regulations.

Marney Walker is an independent occupational therapist specializing in advising on the design of inclusive and accessible housing. She has a combination of experience in housing and social care, training in design, and teaching about disability and society. Her current research at Lab4Living, Sheffield Hallam University, explores how design can support the expression of everyday aesthetic preferences.

This is an opportunity to highlight the Royal College of Occupational Therapists (RCOT) Specialist Section – Housing as a source of support and information. It is noteworthy that of the contributors listed above, eight are or have been members, with most having served on the section's National Executive Committee.

Acknowledgements

All books require cooperation, communication and support from a wide range of people, not just those listed as contributors, and this one is no different. We would like to acknowledge and thank our families, colleagues and Jessica Kingsley Publishers, for their support, tolerance and patience as we have worked on this project. We would also like to thank Amrit Ryatt, Penny Lawrence, Fiona Lillycrop and Jenny Streather.

Introduction

A form of housing is, for most people, 'home', although the place we live in may not meet our needs as our situation changes. As families grow and reduce in size, we may move to larger properties or downsize to reflect the change. When our ability to complete occupations we need or want to do is impaired by barriers within our homes, there is a need to resolve or remove these to promote independence or facilitate care provision.

As occupational therapists working in social care, housing and independent practice, we provide the advice, support and recommendations to adapt properties to meet people's changing needs. Our ability to balance the **medical and social models of disability** is our unique selling point (USP), placing us in a strong position to assess areas of need and to identify barriers within the home environment that cause or exacerbate these. This reflects the **Person-Environment-Occupation-Performance (PEOP) model** of practice (Baum, Christiansen and Bass 2015), and enables us to promote effective multi-professional cross-disciplinary casework, often with the occupational therapist as the central hub in a communication network.

The occupational therapy profession's strength is our holistic approach, encompassing the physical, emotional and social aspects of a person's life, enabling us to understand not only why there is an area of need, but also how that affects the person's mental health and wellbeing. This presents a challenge for those designing occupational therapy courses – how to fit in all the possible permutations of knowledge and information required by qualified practitioners. This challenge is brought into focus in social care, where occupational therapists are expected to be 'specialist-generalists', developing a depth of knowledge across a number of specialist areas including moving and handling, postural management, prescription of **equipment**...and **adaptations**.

This book is designed to support your entry into this area of practice. It is not intended to replace the 'on the job' learning from discussions with or observations of colleagues, or the osmotic process of assimilating knowledge just by being around others working in the same area of practice. Nor does it replace more formal learning opportunities, be these face-to-face or online. The intention is to provide a firm foundation for practice, supporting you as you acquire knowledge and experience. It is a practical, solution-based resource that may provide the answers you are looking for, or if not, signpost you to where that may be found.

All pages marked ★ and the accompanying videos can be downloaded from https://library.jkp.com/redeem using the code EDKQQWA. Keeping a notebook handy will help you make the most of this book and the online resources.

Words and phrases highlighted in bold at their first mention are included in the glossary of terms at the back of the book.

1

The Meaning of Home

Knowledge check

Before you dive into this book, take a step back and consider your own home:

* What is it about your home that is important to you?

* How does it make you feel?

* Is it the physical building, an emotional connection, or the things contained within the building?

Write your thoughts down – aim for about 450 words – and then, when you have completed this, highlight three key words that summarize how you feel.

You may have been slightly surprised opening this book to find that this first activity is a reflection on how you feel about your own home. Surely this book aims to provide practical hints, tips and ideas on the adaptations process in *other* people's homes?

It is important to remember that at the centre of any recommendation is the person being supported, and that what you are recommending may have a significant impact on their life. Still you ask: why me and my home? If you haven't taken the time to complete your reflection, please do have a go and put your thoughts down on paper. Hopefully you will then recognize the depths of attachment you have to that place you call 'home'. Also, by considering the notes you have made and then selecting three keywords, you may realize that these are 'of the moment', and that other aspects noted may have been, or will become, more significant as time passes.

This chapter was written in early 2022. After two years of pandemic and lockdowns your view of home may have changed. Working from home, perhaps isolated from the place identified as home, or coming to a realization that your home configuration no longer 'works' may affect your view of home. We like living in spaces furnished to reflect our tastes and preferences with a view of green space. We don't like working from inside our homes needing a sense of separation between home and work. For many these reflections will have brought to the forefront changing thoughts and feelings about a place often taken for granted.

Within the context of this book, why does this matter? Is it important that we have realized that the memories associated with this particular house, for example, aren't attached to its physical structure? The simple answer is yes, because as occupational therapists (and other professionals) recommending and making changes to the homes of those you are supporting, it is vital that you appreciate the impact of your decision-making on people's needs and preferences.

Before we move on to chapters on more practical matters, we'd like to explore the meaning of home in a little more depth, as in this there may be aspects you recognize from your own reflections. The space we call 'home' has different levels of meaning – some physical, and some linked to non-tangible aspects of life (Fox Mahoney 2007). Are the 'bricks and mortar' your 'home', or is a sense of 'home' created by the things (and people) within that structure? Alternatively, is it the emotional attachment and feelings associated with all of these that make us relate to somewhere as being our home? For us, the approach taken by Kylén *et al.* (2019), proposing that 'housing' is different to 'home', makes sense: 'housing' is the physical space or building, and 'home' relates to the meanings and personal experience attached to it. For most, these two are intertwined and interconnected, although you may disagree.

While the emotional connection we feel to home may appear focused on the security we derive from the space, there are other aspects to consider (Clutton, Grisbooke and Pengelly 2006). For many there is the financial investment associated with home ownership – and not just for those who own their home. The decisions we make about what we place within our homes are not only to meet a practical need. Where we can, we curate these spaces with items that are both useful and provide pleasure or satisfaction, or through our choice of décor. This ability to choose some of what we surround ourselves with provides us with a sense of control.

Our homes provide us with comfort, as a representation of ourselves to those who visit, and also a choice in how we spend our income. For some these decisions may be impulsive, while for others, consideration of the implications of planned changes may require reflection, either due to the emotional impact of changes to a key space or due to the financial outlay required. A new kitchen might be considered a practicality where, as long as there is sufficient storage and work surfaces, the colour of the doors and trim has little relevance. For others their decision-making will be influenced by the emotions associated with meal preparation and time spent with loved ones – the ambience of the space as important as practicality.

Burrell (2014, cited in Visser 2019) considers the occupations linked to homemaking as contributing to our desire to have control over our living space. Després (1991) views 'home' as a symbol of achievement and control as well as self-expression and somewhere we have freedom of action. As occupational therapists we should recognize and enable the ability to engage in homemaking and household activities as these contribute to physical and emotional wellbeing. Després (1991) describes home as being a sanctuary, something that evolves over time, linked to what is familiar and providing us with a feeling of belonging. Beyond the physical there are other key aspects associated with the place we call home. Dovey (1985) advises that these have triple value: social, psychological and cultural.

The financial investments we make in choosing and creating our homes are not the only ones linked to its physical entity. The location or setting of a home provides us with connections and continuity. Our home serves as a concrete or physical reference point, which Kylén *et al.* (2019) highlight as a 'place of departure and return', rooting us within our communities. This could be a community in which someone has always lived, or one that provides familiarity. Consider time spent away from your home when on holiday, or a time when you have relocated to a new town or city. Returning home from holiday is often associated with a sense of grounding – you have enjoyed the novel experiences of a different place or culture, but returning home provides a different sense of pleasure.

If you have ever relocated to an unfamiliar place, there can be a disconnect from your environment until you make connections with neighbours and establish your routines. Here, the sense of home is intertwined with your belongings and their associated memories, as well as developing connections to and within the community you are now part of. For some the idea of being in a culturally diverse community will be something they relish, whereas for others they may need the security of being able to access familiar spaces and facilities, and even ingredients or foods.

Where you are considering the feasibility of adapting a space and proposing rehousing as an option, this key connection to a space, place and community and the impact of severing this cannot be underestimated.

Although our purpose as occupational therapists is often to enable occupations through changes to the environment, the socio-emotional aspects of this are, in many ways, greater than the physical ones. Campo *et al.* (2020, p.299) describe home as a 'familiar yet complex concept of great personal and social significance'. Participants interviewed by Bougdah and Salman (2018) described their feelings around home using words that were charged with meanings, with one participant referring to their home as the 'meanings and associations' linked to it rather than the physical space. Similar to Campo *et al.*'s description of home as 'a repository of memories', the participants indicated that they carry the immaterial with them when away from the physical place. This emotional link provides a sense of home for those with more nomadic lifestyles, such as those who move frequently for work or from Gypsy or Traveller communities. They emphasized that home has meaning over and beyond the physical structure of a building. In summarizing what home meant to the participants, Bougdah and Salman (2018) included over 30 different words, evidencing the intensity of the personal experience for the person.

Considering these views as well as the occupational therapist's role in the adaptations process, we recognize the need for home to be a place of 'ease and comfort' (Campo *et al.* 2020). Adaptations are recommended to enable activities that have become difficult through a person's changing health or abilities. We also need to remember that home is a place for meaningful occupations – as Kylén *et al.* (2019) note, home is linked to a sense of purpose.

As we age, the ability for us to remain in our own home may be affected. Although adaptations are needed at any age, Gustafson (2014, cited in Kylén *et al.* 2019) advises that the majority of older people want to 'age in place'. Kylén *et al.* (2019) note that we cannot presume that preferences expressed by previous generations reflect today's values. The ageing process includes transitioning from work to retirement, for example, a significant change that requires ongoing identity negotiation (Kylén *et al.* 2019). It is worth noting that any significant change, including those linked to changes in physical or mental health, also requires the person to internally re-evaluate their own identity. This may include consideration of what is wanted or needed in a person's home.

There are some differences between the meaning of home for adults and for children, adults appearing to refer more to spatial control and social supervision, and children linking home with freedom of action alongside physical and emotional security (Després 1991). In discussions with child participants, Campo *et al.* (2020) noted that initial responses linked home to a more concrete entity – somewhere for physical possessions; further exploration also identified the emotional weight associated with a child's home.

This brief summary on the meaning of home can only be a superficial overview. It is important that as professionals you remember the weight and value that home has for the person and their family: a 'place for continuity' (Kylén *et al.* 2019, p.308); 'a complex interplay of space, relationships, the body, and time' (Visser 2019, p.7); and 'an integral part of the way people experience their dwelling environment' (Bougdah and Salman 2018, p.712). Remember that home 'is not a static unchanging concept' (Visser 2019, p.7), and that although you are asking people to make changes to a space with value and importance, these are designed to enhance their quality of life, promote their independence and enable choice.

2

What Is a Home Adaptation?

Knowledge check

Adaptations vary from person to person and between locations and level of need. Pick an area from the list below, and write down as many adaptations as you can (ideally aim for six) that would be needed to promote occupations there:

* Outside space

* Moving between different levels in the home (e.g., ground to first floor, internal steps)

* Bathroom

* Kitchen

(Please retain this list, as you will need it later. But for those who can't wait, see Table 1 at the end of this chapter!)

This chapter clarifies what we mean by 'home adaptation' and the difference between this and items of equipment. It introduces the approach recommended in *Adaptations without Delay* (RCOT 2019), a **Royal College of Occupational Therapists (RCOT)** publication that challenges the 'traditional' approach of 'minor' or 'major' adaptations, and the implications of this on current practice.

Our first question is, what exactly is an 'adaptation'? Let us look at some definitions to help. The NHS (2022) defines home adaptations as 'changes you can make to your home that make it safer and easier to move around and do everyday tasks'. From this definition we can say with some certainty that in line with Ainsworth and de Jonge (2011), an adaptation is a physical alteration to a home with the purpose of increasing safety and promoting independence for daily occupations of both necessity and choice.

When is it an 'adaptation' and when is it 'equipment'?

We are accustomed to using the words 'adaptation' and 'equipment', as we believe we know what they mean when prescribing them to support people to overcome occupational barriers. Adaptations are usually made to the fabric of a building and are generally a permanent alteration; in certain circumstances they can be temporary. Equipment is usually a product or device that a person uses to interact with the built environment that assists with carrying out activities of daily living; equipment can be freestanding or fixed to the fabric of the building.

There isn't a generally accepted definition of equipment or adaptations, and the interpretation of what they constitute can vary from locality to locality, which has consequences for funding and provision. An example of a product that may be considered as both equipment and an adaptation is a **tracked hoist**, which can be funded via an adaptations grant or by social care. Tracked hoists are subject to the *Provision and Use of Work Equipment Regulations 1998 (PUWER)* (HSE 2022) and *Lifting Operations and Lifting Equipment Regulations (LOLER) 1998* (HSE 1999). This is a complex topic, because which regulations apply depends on who uses and owns the tracked hoist. Where the tracked hoist is provided via an adaptations grant, the hoist is the property of the grant recipient, and they have a responsibility under LOLER regulations to ensure it is in good working order. On the other hand, if an employed caregiver uses the tracked hoist, then the employer has responsibilities under both PUWER and LOLER regulations to ensure it is in safe working order and appropriate training on its operation is provided.

Terminology

You will most likely be familiar with the terms 'housing adaptation' and 'home modification'. These terms are often used interchangeably and may convey different meanings depending where in the world you practice. In the UK the term 'home' or 'housing adaptation' is used to describe the physical alteration of a **property** to meet the needs of a person living with a **disability** (NHS 2022), while the term 'home modification' is more commonly used in the USA, Canada and Australia.

Wahl *et al.* (2009, p.357) suggest that home modifications are 'efforts to improve a given physical home environment with the aim to address the functional needs of a person.' Fänge and Iwarsson (2005, p.45) suggest home modifications are: 'The alteration of permanent physical features in the home environment, i.e., the objective is to reduce the demands of the physical environment on the home and its close surroundings, in order to enhance daily activities, and promote the ability to lead an independent life'.

Another issue that is commonly raised is using the term **Disabled Facilities Grant (DFG)** to refer to a significant home adaptation. This is problematic as a DFG is actually the means or the process by which facilities are provided or funded. It is better to use 'home adaptation' as a catch-all phrase, as this covers all options. Also, a DFG is only available in England, Wales and Northern Ireland, with Scotland having their own system, although Wales does have some divergence in the DFG process compared to England where certain types of housing associations are concerned. Chapter 6 provides information on the differences between the four home nations.

Tracked hoists provide a perfect example of using the appropriate terminology when prescribing interventions. 'Ceiling tracked', 'overhead', 'wall-mounted' and 'gantry hoist' are all terms that are used interchangeably to describe a hoist that is attached to the fabric of the building.

The other aspect of describing a tracked hoist is the track layout. For example, what is the difference between an 'H track' and an 'XY track'? There are several ways to interpret these descriptions. 'H track' may describe the movement of the hoist on its track, but does this mean that it has two separate straight tracks with a connecting track – for example, where one track is in the bedroom and the second is in the bathroom and the two are connected? Or does it describe two parallel pieces of track connected by a crossbeam that allows the hoist to be positioned at any point within a defined area?

This illustrates where terminology may cause confusion and miscommunication, as your interpretation may differ from another person's.

Let us look at how we might categorize home adaptations. The RCOT (2019) suggests that adaptations fit into three distinct categories: universal, targeted and specific. The next question to answer is, how do we define these categories?

- *Universal:* These include adaptations that are beneficial to all people and may already be part of the building, for example a handrail on an exterior set of steps. Another interpretation of 'universal' is adaptations that are identified by the person who requires them and that are not assessed for or prescribed by a practitioner.

- *Targeted:* This refers to where a person's circumstances are routine or generally straightforward, although the person needs support to find a solution. Here the adaptation is likely to be assessed for and prescribed by a practitioner in collaboration with the person. The adaptation could be a relatively standard adaptation, either structural or non-structural.

- *Specific:* This is where the person's circumstances are complex and they have many differing requirements. In this case the solution requires detailed assessment and prescription by an expert practitioner, and the adaptation is likely to be highly personalized, and structural or non-structural.

The Welsh Government (2019) takes an alternative approach, suggesting in *Housing Adaptations Service Standards* that adaptations could be described in the following categories:

- *Small:* Inexpensive adaptations that can be provided quickly and that do not require building or planning approval; these may have been assessed by a practitioner.

- *Medium:* Adaptations that do not require building or planning approval; these may be structural and are likely to be assessed by a suitably qualified person.

- *Large:* Adaptations that require significant structural alterations or highly specialist adaptations; adaptations that fall in this category will require building or planning approval and assessment by an occupational therapist.

Comparing the two lists we see that they align. The Welsh Government's descriptions assist both practitioners and non-practitioners to understand the scale and complexity of recommendations – they offer alternative wording for use when discussing options with non-professionals or those outside of the housing sector.

Another area of terminology that can be problematic is the description of the item or facility you are recommending. This can be summed up by the 'toilet seat and frame debate' – do you use a generic term or a manufacturer's branding (like 'vacuum cleaner' and 'Hoover', which are synonymous)? Other examples include using the manufacturer's name for a wash and dry toilet and the interchangeable use of shower or changing stretcher (or bench).

Consider the images that the terms 'level access shower' and 'wet room' conjure up. If someone expects a fully tiled wet room and 'simply' has the bath replaced, the adaptation is unlikely to match their expectation.

We can't give a full list of terminology here, but do be mindful of the descriptors you use. There is a need for both clarity and consistency. You will be making recommendations, adding to case notes, requesting quotes and having discussions with those involved. Slipping between different descriptors raises the possibility of a misunderstanding.

> One thing to remember is that adaptations take many forms, but occupational therapists are required to consider best use of the available space before considering adaptations that extend the existing property.

The discussion on the meaning of 'home' leads to the way an adaption is designed: its appearance does not have to be clinical or institutional. Good design takes into account aesthetics, **accessibility** and Inclusive and Universal Design, resulting in a space or facility that meets the needs of the person and all those in their household.

This chapter has briefly introduced housing adaptations and two approaches to replace the 'traditional' 'minor' and 'major' descriptors. The information within this book reflects this current approach and has highlighted a need to consider the terminology adopted when completing recommendations.

Remember your list of adaptations from the activity at the start of this chapter? Here is our list – but there will be more:

Table 1. List of possible adaptations

Outside space	Transfer between different levels	Bathroom	Kitchen
Dropped kerb	Grab rail	Lever taps	Task lighting
Hardstanding	Stair rail	Sensor taps	Cupboard handle design
Path	Surface finish	Lighting control	Lowered work surface
Ramp	Lighting	Task lighting	Height-adjustable work surface
Railings	Platform lift	Type of bath	Shallow sink
Grab rail	Stairlift	Wall-hung basin	Lever taps
Lighting	Through floor lift	Height-adjustable basin	Sensor taps
Fencing	Ramp	Level-access shower	Height-adjustable cupboard
Gate	Highlight stair nosing	Slip-resistant floor finish	Power sockets
Entry system		Shower type	Gas shut off switch
		Flush mechanism	Switched stopcock
		Switched stopcock	

3

The Role of the Occupational Therapist in Home Adaptations

Knowledge check

Here are some questions for you to reflect on:

* Are occupational therapists essential in the successful completion of an adaptation?

* Considering your list of adaptations from the previous chapter, which of these requires the involvement of an occupational therapist?

Occupational therapists work in diverse settings with a variety of roles and remits, all contributing to the 'bigger picture' supporting positive outcomes. Addressing the 'imbalance caused by the ageing process or disability within the home environment, occupational therapists are seen as the experts in this field of practice' (Russell, Ormerod and Newton 2018, p.1). Traditionally we see occupational therapists in social care, housing and independent practice as leading in this field, although there are many more occupational therapy roles that contribute to successful schemes.

Where do occupational therapists become involved?
Alongside traditional housing and social care roles, occupational therapists are well placed to influence new-build property designs, and in a housing role, the review and refurbishment of existing stock. In the independent

sector occupational therapists have the freedom to work with individuals as well as on larger projects.

> A case in point – new-build properties have the potential to be accessible in a less overt way through 'designing out' the need for later adaptation through extending accessibility beyond level thresholds and wider doorways on the ground floor. Perhaps if they included occupational therapists in the design of new-builds...?

When do occupational therapists get involved?

The earlier the better! Involvement at the initiation of a project or housing stock review enables occupational therapists to 'design in accessibility', identifying barriers and promoting **Inclusive Design** in a way that doesn't highlight 'disability'. For casework, early involvement provides the time to work with the person to understand their situation, abilities, needs and preferences before recommending an adaptation.

Why do occupational therapists get involved?

Occupational therapists have a unique skill set. You understand both the medical and social model of disability, and the impact of medical conditions and disability on the person and their family. **Holistic assessments** identify strengths and areas of need in the context of the individual and those supporting them.

Assessment

Your assessments and interventions are completed in the home environment, enabling the assimilation of information, assessment and observations, synthesizing this with the environment in which the person lives. This, with your knowledge of property types, construction methods and adaptations, informs your recommendations.

> Your role is not so much as 'expert', but rather to use your expertise and knowledge to inform and support the adaptation process. No profession stands still; new approaches evolve and will inform your work.

For those in housing adaptations, *Adaptations without Delay* (RCOT 2019) refreshes your approach and language. For example, the move away from 'minor' and 'major' adaptations to 'universal', 'targeted' and 'specialist' provides an empowering approach.

The role you are employed in directs the extent of your involvement in adaptations. Although we can't list specifics, as teams and services differ widely, your understanding of the role and remit of occupational therapists is important as these provide firm foundations for practice. Overstepping boundaries means that you are working without authority, and risk damaging essential working relationships. The most important working relationship you have is with the person you are supporting. You should aim for **co-production**, emphasizing the equality of all involved, working together to achieve an outcome.

Co-production

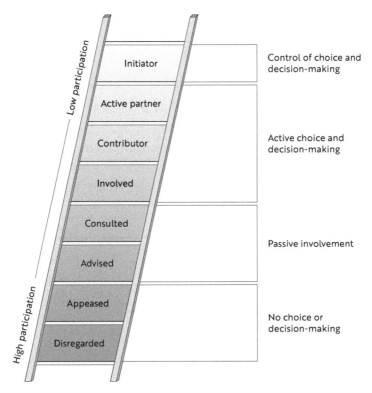

FIGURE 1. DEGREES OF SERVICE USER PARTICIPATION IN THE ADAPTATION PROCESS
Source: Ruth Parker (2019)

Co-production is a joint enterprise, but it doesn't happen without taking a proactive approach, as those you are supporting may expect you to lead and make key decisions on their behalf. Reflect on your role in the adaptation process and how you work with those you are supporting. To achieve this, consider the 'Ladder of children's participation' (Hart 1992), placing this in the context of housing adaptations and the way you work with people. Figure 1 provides a model to reflect on your approach to co-production.

Co-production
Working from the foot of the ladder upwards:

- *Disregarded or appeased:* At no point should you act in this way! Be aware that others may adopt this stance, making decisions on behalf of a family member or **tenant**. It is not done with a negative intent; it is because they believe they are acting in the person's best interests.

- *Advised or consulted:* Here you would still be adopting an approach that acts 'for' rather than 'with' a person. You are deciding what is most appropriate, and either telling them or presenting a curated list of options. The person remains a passive partner in the process.

- *Involved, contributor or active partner:* You are now actively involving those you work with. They have a voice and can influence the outcome of discussions.

- *Initiator:* This is when you play second string and the person leads; they are empowered, and you are there in a supporting role.

What does this mean in the real world? We can't presume people have the energy or capacity to be initiators. And as with any ladder, we will ascend and descend. (We recommend missing the bottom two rungs, but for physical ladders, safety first – these are essential!) The process of moving up and down through the rungs of the ladder has variables. If someone tells you they need (or want) an adaptation, they are active in the process. If you are introducing the idea of home adaptation and they have not considered it, you start in an advisory role. From this you move on to more active co-production.

Not all decisions and actions sit on the same rung; you may be sent a scheme that in your professional opinion does not meet identified needs, creating more barriers than it resolves. What is the appropriate response? Do you sit with the person and discuss every point in detail? We would advise not – it may raise expectations and muddy the waters, as well as taking up valuable time (theirs and yours). In this scenario the *advisory* rung is probably appropriate. You can advise that you have reviewed the scheme, and it didn't meet the identified needs so you have sent it back with comments.

Reviewing a scheme that is practical and addresses the identified barriers enables you to move into active choice and decision-making. You still move between the rungs, but here your role is supportive rather than leading. You may drop back into 'advising' – Building Regulations and legislation mean that not everything is negotiable. Active conversations around the reasons for this aid understanding. Be aware of the approach you are taking at any point in the process, and reflect and adjust as needed.

Do we ever encounter an initiator? This person would be someone who decides that they want to adapt their home, finds a surveyor and contractor, and then chooses finishes, fixtures and fittings. Given this level of active involvement, would they need an occupational therapist? You can still be involved, providing advice and information to support their decisions, guiding design choices to promote accessibility and independence.

Assessment completion is addressed in more detail in Chapter 7 on key skills, but it is the starting point of any intervention, informing you of the person's situation, barriers and **enablers**. Your role is one of active listening and appreciative inquiry, asking the 'right' questions. Pro formas give a structure for recording and reporting information; your questions and the answers they elicit determine the quality of the evidence guiding your actions (see the Appendix).

The assessment leads to identification and agreement of objectives. Without these you cannot proceed with casework or recommend adaptations. Clear objectives with realistic outcomes are the base of your involvement, and assist all involved with understanding what is being worked towards.

Professional reasoning

A key aspect of your role is to evidence your reasoning. Chapter 5 on professional reasoning may not be why you opened this book, but please don't skip it. Where there is disagreement on action or outcome, or uncertainty on what is to be achieved, evidencing and articulating thought processes provides clarity. **Professional reasoning** enables you to demonstrate the wider impact of your recommendations. For example:

- *Ramps:* Simply providing access to the home? No, it is enabling access to the wider community, and all the benefits associated with that.

- *Kitchen adaptations:* Simply enabling meal preparation? No, nutrition is key to good health, independence and choice as well as mental and physical wellbeing.

Signposting and advice

The role of occupational therapists is also to provide advice and information. This enables people to make choices and be proactive in decision-making. Signposting is not 'fobbing off' someone to avoid adding to a busy caseload; ensuring a person is directed to the appropriate service, support or source of guidance demonstrates you understand your role and remit, and recognize that you cannot be all things to all people.

Advice includes health promotion, although it can be argued that this was not previously a developed part of the occupational therapy role. Good health is a facilitator, and if you can prevent or remove barriers arising from health conditions, then you have a role to play. The Allied Health Professions Federation has published a framework that demonstrates the value of health promotion (Hindle and Charlesworth 2019). The RCOT website has resources for members on this aspect of practice including falls prevention, a key area where the home environment can be adapted to reduce risks during mobilization and transfers.[1]

While we must reduce risk, we must not be risk-averse. Gallagher (2013) advises that engagement in everyday lives requires an element of risk-taking, challenging us to move beyond a negative view of risk, and recognizing that it offers opportunity. Where you are facilitating positive and informed risk-taking, consider how this affects those you are working with – people and families. Providing your rationale and risk evaluation for a scenario enables understanding of the objectives and outcomes you are promoting. This also demonstrates that you have considered risks and are supporting action(s) and choice safely.

Occupational therapists do not just assess and recommend adaptations; they prescribe equipment to support and enable occupations. A key aspect of the role is to ensure that the two responsibilities are coordinated. First, that the adaptation has the space and construction to enable equipment to be installed and used as intended, and second, any equipment delivery is timed with adaptation completion as far as possible. There is nothing more frustrating than having an adaptation such as a level-access shower completed, but unusable, as the shower bench, hoist or shower chair has not been delivered.

There are aspects of adaptations where you will be working with experts in their field, and times when you will have the higher level of knowledge. Identify when you need to lead from the front, where your experience is key to meeting objectives. In these instances, you may call in equipment

---

1   See www.rcot.co.uk/practice-resources/occupational-therapy-topics/public-health

provider reps to assist, such as with modular ramps or tracked hoists. You will need their expertise in how these work within the space, but be mindful that they don't take a lead on what objectives should be met. There is a balance that needs to be maintained. For direct discussions around the **usability** and suitability of designs in facilitating occupations; reps bring a depth of knowledge about the equipment they provide, but you understand the barriers a person has faced, the way they live (and want to live), and the potential for equipment and adaptations to remove barriers.

The information in this chapter (and in this book) highlights the role of occupational therapists as communicators and coordinators. More to the point, you can view yourself as a communication hub, one that provides advice and information as well as facilitating information-sharing between people, families, caregivers and a wide range of professionals.

This is not to say that occupational therapists provide a project management role, or that communication can only be passed via you. It may be that as an occupational therapist in independent practice you take on a case management role, of which housing adaptation forms a part. In general, project management of an adaptation will sit with a building professional. Identifying when you should or shouldn't act as a communication hub helps you empower people, promoting their choice and control in the adaptation process. You communicate the necessary information to ensure a scheme will address identified needs and facilitate understanding of the impact of barriers. Your assessments allow you to interpret a proposed scheme and predict effectiveness through discussions with the person, surveyor (or equivalent) and contractor.

One area to ponder – should occupational therapists be the bearer of bad news? Not all recommendations progress to adaptation. Should you advise the person of this decision? We argue that this is not within the role and remit of occupational therapists. The decision to decline a submitted recommendation is made by the local or housing authority, and they are best placed to explain their decision and the next steps, such as appealing the decision.

Different areas and teams work in different ways, and there is no one-size-fits-all guide to roles and remits. *Adaptations without Delay* (RCOT 2019), 'Disabled Facilities Grant (DFG) delivery: Guidance for local authorities in

England' (HM Government 2022) and the design and construction process protocol proposed by Russell *et al.* (2018) offer some guidance, however.

This chapter has provided a broad outline of the role and remit of the occupational therapist working in housing adaptations. You may work purely in a housing sector, or in social care, with a wider remit for intervention. The key to success in either area is to understand the parameters of your team's scope, as this provides a focus for your interventions and a foundation for practice.

The questions posed at the start of the chapter may seem strange in a book promoting the contribution occupational therapists bring to the adaptation process. Occupational therapists have their role to play, but this includes enabling those you support to be proactive and make choices. An awareness of this, alongside that of your role and remit, means that you can focus on supporting those who require your assistance, either through a need for advocacy and guidance, or due to the complexity of the adaptation required.

4

Key People in the Adaptations Process

ELIZABETH COOPER

The process of adapting a person's home requires support and cooperation across professionals and disciplines. It is perhaps the area of occupational therapy practice with the greatest scope for working with professionals who do not have a medical background. Those working in this area of practice have the opportunity to contribute to the delivery and further development of housing services (Ainsworth and de Jonge 2011), and therefore a recognition of all those contributing to housing adaptations is of benefit. This chapter highlights some of the key persons contributing to this area of practice.

The person

The person who has been referred for an assessment depending on your work setting may be referred to as a service user client or patient. They are at the centre of everything occupational therapists do.

Family

The impact of an adaptation on any other family member in the household must be considered. There may be other adults or children in the house with or without a disability, which may influence the proposed adaptation. Older or vulnerable people may be supported by family members who are not resident with them.

Occupational therapists

Occupational therapists in housing and social care have specialist experience and knowledge of assessment, prescription and recommending of specialist equipment and adaptations for individuals to live more easily and safely in their own homes. Other occupational therapists contributing to decision-making for adaptations include those working in hospitals, wheelchair services and independent practice.

Grants officer

(Titles vary depending on the authority and job role, so we have used a generic title here.) Grants officers provide members of the public with general advice about the options available, as per the authority's housing grants assistance policy, to support in:

- Maintaining independence.

- Managing DFG applications, as per the local authorities Housing Grants Assistance Policy, in line with the Housing Grants, Construction and Regeneration Act 1996, and for Discretionary Assistance, as per Regulatory Reform Order 2002.

- Assisting with the application process and provision of supporting documentation, including financial information.

- Producing schematic drawings using computer-aided design (CAD) software or contracting out external services where required, to complete **architectural drawings.**

- Preparing the schedule of work and specifications.

- Consulting with the occupational therapist to ensure proposed works are necessary and appropriate.

Housing officer

Housing officers are usually responsible for a particular estate or group of properties. The role involves supporting tenants and encouraging them to take part in tenancy groups that help shape the community in which they live. They assess the needs of people applying for housing, and carry out regular inspections to make sure all properties are in a good state of repair, dealing with anti-social behaviour and broken tenancy agreements, referring tenants to appropriate sources of benefits and welfare advice.

Technical officer

Technical officers are responsible for advising on the feasibility of adaptations in social housing, drawing up schemes and overseeing works.

Surveyor

The surveyor undertakes surveys to establish design types and the structural conditions of properties, preparing drawings of existing properties and adaptation proposals using CAD software. They prepare designs from feasibility through to final design proposals, and detailed schedules of work and specifications, ensuring relevant regulations and legislation are complied with. They closely monitor the completion of works, including the agreement to any variations, and authorize payments when due. If employed by a local authority, they undertake the role of lead officer on delivering adaptations, including the coordination of other disciplines within the design, administration and inspection of projects.

Architect

Architects create designs for new construction projects, alterations and redevelopment. They can remove potential **barriers** for those people with disabilities, and promote ease of access for everybody.

Architectural technician

Architectural technicians create building designs using CAD, offer technical guidance and liaise with construction design teams, either as part of a local authority social housing team or with architects or surveyors.

Home Improvement Agency

Home Improvement Agency (HIA) services originated over 30 years ago to work with low-income, older owner-occupiers with a vision to provide responsive client-centred solutions for home repair, maintenance and adaptation problems. The early pioneers, independent 'Care and Repair' or 'Staying Put' services, were small-scale and largely funded by the charitable sector. While many of the original agencies still operate, most agencies are now managed by housing associations, local authorities or private companies, with funding from local authorities and health services.

The HIA sector is almost as well defined by its differences as by its similarities, but all HIAs share two key facets:

- Client-centred support provided in a person's home.

- Expertise in making changes to the physical fabric of the home.

Planning department

Planning permission will be needed for:

- A new-build property.

- Making a major change to a building, such as an extension.

- Changing the use of the building.

- Alterations to a listed building or some building works in conservation areas.

Building control

This department covers Building Regulations, minimum standards for design, construction and alterations to buildings. The building control officer issues approval to start building work, completion certificates, inspecting and carrying out surveys of potentially dangerous buildings and approving demolitions. They also check:

- Fire precautions and requirements (even for a small extension).

- Ventilation to rooms and roof voids, waste, roof coverings and insulation, staircases, safety glazing.

- Excavations for foundations, damp proof course and drainage and insulation.

Note that Building Regulations approval is different from planning permission, and both might be needed for some adaptations.

Contractor

Contractors are a crucial part of the adaptation process. Many local authorities have an approved list of contractors, who will deliver quality works in a timely manner, with due consideration of the disabled person and their family. This may be linked to set prices for specified works, which simplifies the tender process.

Landlord

Permission is required from the landlord to carry out any building works or installation of equipment to the rented property. This applies to both social landlords and privately rented properties.

Equipment provider representative

Equipment provider representatives are usually referred to as the 'equipment rep'. They can provide advice on specialist equipment and offer trials of equipment where appropriate. Liaising with reps supports the adaptation process, and coordination between equipment orders and building works enables the person to make full use of their new facility on completion. Neighbours must be informed if the building work is on the boundary between the properties or on an existing party wall or party structure, or digging below and near to the foundation level of their property. Building works can be quite disruptive, so occupational therapists need to be aware of the impact this may have on neighbours.

This chapter is only a brief introduction to the main cast of characters involved in the home adaptation process, and we are sure you will be thinking 'but what about x?' Every situation is unique; we will likely meet people outside of this list who will be influential in achieving the outcomes identified for that situation with their role every bit as valuable.

5

Professional Reasoning

Knowledge check

* What is professional reasoning, and how does this differ from clinical reasoning or common sense?

* As a practitioner, how do you evidence professional reasoning in practice?

Professional reasoning may appear a dry topic when we can be making recommendations that will have a visible impact on the lives of those we are working with. Bear with us for a short while as we explain what it is in relation to home adaptations, and how you can evidence this in your record keeping. There is a wealth of literature around this topic, but rather than provide references for each and every point made, we will limit these to key points or quotes.

So what is professional reasoning?
Interchangeable phrases are used that all describe the same thought process, including clinical reasoning, clinical judgement, problem-solving, decision-making and critical thinking. This book adopts the term 'professional reasoning' rather than 'clinical reasoning', reflecting the approach by Schell and Schell (2008), as this is more inclusive of the diverse settings occupational therapists practice in outside of clinical settings.

Unsworth and Baker (2016, p.5) describe professional reasoning as a process that 'involves all the thinking processes of the clinician as s/he moves into, through and out of the therapeutic relationship and therapy process with a client'. In your professional role you seek out information, observe situations and environments, assimilating and synthesizing accumulated knowledge to support your decision-making. This goes beyond the decision or course of action you take, encompassing evaluation of outcomes and a process of reflection and learning, moving through to review and re-evaluation.

Professional reasoning provides the structure or framework underpinning the actions, interventions and recommendations you make. This facilitates effective resolution of issues or needs identified through the **assessment** and review process, enabling you to work towards agreed objectives.

As you develop skills, knowledge and experience, your professional reasoning abilities extend and develop, becoming intrinsic to your practice. While you process information and make appropriate decisions in more complex situations, you are required to present these in a manner that can be understood by those you are working with. This communication of ideas and the evidence that supports them will be articulated in different ways between those you are supporting and a wider team of professionals. Your ability to explain your thought processes and decision-making is especially important as you support those entering the occupational therapy profession or those who are new to this area of practice.

Adopting a conscious approach to developing professional reasoning, and actively reflecting on situations and learning opportunities, will enable you to understand how you have reached your conclusions, and supports articulation of those conclusions.

What is the difference between professional reasoning and clinical reasoning?

Having read the previous section, has this altered your answer to the first question posed at the beginning of this chapter? There is no difference really between the two terms, which are used to describe the thought processes that support actions and recommendations. Where there is a difference is with common sense. Yes, many of the actions recommended or suggestions made appear to be basic common sense – note the use of the word 'appear'. In the Collins dictionary 'common sense' is described as: 'Your *common sense* is your natural ability to make good judgments and to behave in a practical and sensible way' (2022).

Yes, your recommendations are (hopefully) all of the above, but what they aren't is based solely on 'natural ability'. You have undertaken a professional qualification that has provided you with the knowledge and ability to complete assessments and observations. These tools combine with knowledge and experience (yours and others'), enabling you to analyse situations based on evidence. From this, you can consider available options that will enable you to recommend the most appropriate action. What to the observer may appear to be 'simply' common sense is, in fact, *well considered evidence-based professional reasoning. This leads us to consider how we complete and articulate professional reasoning.*

The professional reasoning cycle

The occupational therapy process is, in many instances, cyclical, moving from assessment to intervention and then to review, when the process restarts if needed. Levett-Jones *et al.* (2010) created an image of the clinical reasoning cycle for student nurses. This provides an effective structure for the occupational therapy adaptation process, and we have utilized this to demonstrate progression through initial contact, recommendation, adaptation and on to review of the completed adaptation (see Figure 2).

1. Beginning at the 12 o'clock position, start by *considering the person's situation*. You are all familiar with the different sources of information available, but one point to remember is to ensure informed consent is in place – you cannot presume the person is happy for you to contact others who may be supporting them.

    So where do you get your information from? Documentation/ multi-disciplinary team.

    Referral documents: These will tell you what the referrer *thinks* is needed as well as (hopefully) giving you background information about the person, their household and the property.

    Previous involvements: Past case notes will include information such as previous abilities and discussions held. These can be used for comparison once you have completed the assessment.

    Other professionals: If you have been given consent to contact others involved with the person, this can be an opportunity to widen your understanding of the situation. This isn't to say contact everyone, but gathering more information about the person's medical condition and understanding the impact of any treatment programmes or prognosis will support your decision-making.

    Family members: This could be because the referral is for a child, or because the person requires an advocate or support.

    The person: This is the focus of your initial assessment or reassessment, providing details of the person's needs and abilities, their wants and preferences and their expectations.

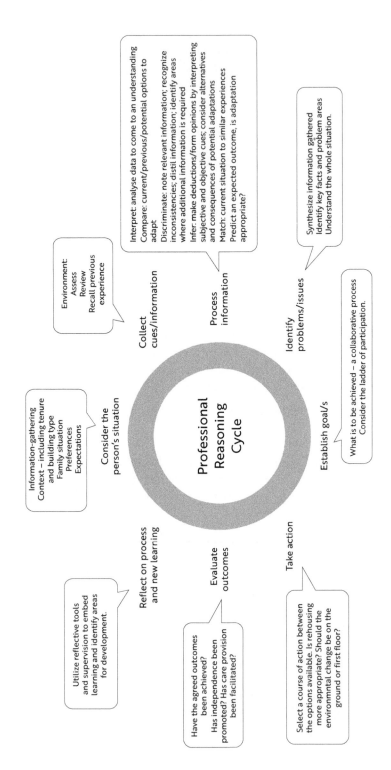

FIGURE 2. PROFESSIONAL REASONING CYCLE FOR HOUSING ADAPTATIONS
Source: Ruth Parker, adapted from Levett-Jones et al. (2010)

2. Moving clockwise, the next step is to look at the environment and collect *cues*. You have assessed the person and now you are looking at how the environment provides enablers and barriers. Review these in light of your perception of the person's situation, recalling relevant knowledge that supports your understanding. This includes knowledge of the person's medical condition(s), legislation, construction methods and types of equipment you might consider prescribing.

3. Having gathered information, you need to *process* what you have learned, interpreting the information, comparing the current and previous situations and considering what can be achieved. This process requires you to filter the information, discarding what is not relevant and prioritizing key details. From this you can make deductions and form your opinions of the situation. Matching what you have learned with what you know from past experience will enable you to look at options available, and you can begin to identify an appropriate outcome.

4. Drawing together information and your analysis will enable you to *identify problems and issues*. Within housing adaptations this could be linked to the person or those they live with, the construction of the property, processes or funding. The previous steps in the cycle enable you to be in a position where you can synthesize the information, considering the situation holistically.

5. The next step is familiar within the occupational therapy process: you must *establish goals*. What are you aiming to achieve? Achievable goals or objectives are then developed co-productively. Yes, aspiration is good, but buildings, finance and other aspects of adaptations do limit what can be achieved. For example, increasing the floor area available in a high-rise flat is not possible. Innovative use of existing space is required to meet agreed outcomes.

6. Now *take action*; initially this is making your recommendation(s) based on all of the steps up until now. Alternatively, your action may be inaction – the information gathered may lead you to conclude that it is not appropriate to proceed with a home adaptation. This part of the process leads to further actions. Having made recommendations, review plans, make adjustments to ensure these achieve the identified outcomes, re-evaluate considering any new information and monitor adaptation progress.

7. Once an adaptation is completed, revisit the objectives by *evaluating outcomes*. Did you achieve what you set out to do? Outcomes must be viewed holistically. If the space or facility provided does not enable the occupations of necessity or choice, you cannot say that the outcomes have been effectively achieved.

How do you evidence objectives have been met? Commercial construction projects utilize Post Occupancy Evaluations to ensure that projects meet the design brief. In effect this is what you complete (with less focus on energy efficiency), evaluating the success in promoting occupations.

8. The final step of the professional reasoning process is to *reflect* on what has occurred and what you have learned. This then supports your development and knowledge. Take this through to either a review of this person's situation, or on to the next case you are working on. What does this look like in practice? Table 2 provides examples.

Table 2. Examples of occupational therapy professional reasoning in practice

Process	Description	Example
Consider the person's situation	Referral information	Referral for 40-year-old with a diagnosis of motor neurone disease.
	Previous case note	
	Family situation	Lives with partner, son (12) and daughter (9).
	Type of housing	Owner-occupied terraced house.
	Initial assessment	Identifies bathing and access to first floor as issues.
Collect cues and information	Observation of the home layout/ facilities	No previous adaptations, level access from street, ground floor (GF) bathroom, first floor.
	Barriers and enablers	Bedroom, room for through floor lift.
Process information	Comparison Interpretation Inference	Look at previous involvements, compare changes in ability, consider typical progression of diagnosis, consider impact on family, identify preferred outcome of involvement. Does this meet DFG criteria?

Identify problems/ issues	Synthesize information	What needs addressing? What is the appropriate action? Address access to bathing and to the first floor. GF bathroom can be level-access shower, there is space in the dining room for a through floor lift. How will this affect other family members?
Establish goals	What is to be achieved?	Agree outcomes with person and family: create GF shower room; they request not to proceed with the through floor lift at this time, and want a stairlift in the interim.
Take action	Complete DFG recommendation	Outline issues, confirm long-term need and recommend adaptation(s) to address needs. Monitor the adaptation process, reassess as required if needs change. Consider equipment provision and meet interim needs.
Evaluate	Have outcomes been achieved?	Review the adaptation – have the needs identified at assessment been addressed? Are there any new issues or needs? Can the case be closed to review?
Reflect and review	What went well?	What new knowledge do you have?
New learning	What would you change?	If there were delays, could they have been negated? Is there any good practice you can share?

The professional reasoning cycle takes us through the stages in the process, but also consider the type of influence you will have. Stark *et al.* (2015) advise that this can be categorized as intrinsic or extrinsic.

Intrinsic influences:

- *Impact of the disease or condition:* Although much of what you do in the area of social care or housing is based around your observations and assessment, you understand the lifespan impact of a medical condition or disability. As occupational therapists your USP is your ability to balance the medical and social model of disability. Your interventions consider the lived experience of those you are working with, but your clinical knowledge will enable you to identify future needs.

- *Personal preference:* Completion of a holistic assessment enables you to understand both what a person wants or needs, but also how they would prefer this to be achieved. This guides the recommendations that you make, but make sure that you have listened to and understood the person's point of view, and are certain they have understood the suggestions you have made.

- *Maintenance:* The person's ability to maintain what is provided must be considered. This might be the financial implication of a service contract, or their physical or cognitive ability, now or in the future. This may lead to consideration of interim solutions or ensuring that reviews are scheduled to monitor the situation.

- *Openness to change:* Sometimes you can see an 'ideal' solution, but this may not be received by an open mind. Some people have difficulty in adapting to changes, finding comfort in their routines. Others may find the unknown causes anxiety, especially if this is linked to a financial commitment.

- *Aesthetics:* Our homes say much about us, and for some present the 'face' they want the world to see. If the belief is that a home adaptation such as a ramp will identify them as disabled, it may be that there will be resistance. If adaptations are created following a specification which details finishes that appear clinical rather than reflecting personal taste, this may serve as a daily reminder of disability or lost independence.

Extrinsic influences:

- *Financial aspects:* At the time of writing (2022) the DFG in England is set at a maximum of £30,000, with some local discretion. Recent world events have affected what this amount can provide, placing more people in a position where they may be asked for a contribution to the overall cost. (See Chapter 6 for more details on grant contributions and financial assessments.) For adaptations in social housing this financial pressure has meant that **rehousing** is looked at as an initial option to enable better use of housing stock and budget management.

- *Personal and support networks:* These link to the intrinsic influence of personal preference. What can be offered may require assistance from others, or alternatively, the recommendation may be to support independence. The completion of a holistic assessment will enable you to identify what level of support is in place (or is needed) and reflect this in your adaptation recommendation.

- *Household members:* Changes to meet the needs of one person will often affect those they live with. Your assessment should consider other household members' thoughts, feelings and preferences, and the solutions identified should take these into consideration as far as possible.

- *The property:* The type of property, construction, location and ownership all influence what can be achieved. This book will have given you some understanding of each of these – but there will always be something new or unusual to consider!

Evidencing and recording your professional reasoning

As you become more adept in this area of practice, the decision-making process becomes less overt (and quicker). Developing a higher skill level may mean your 'workings out' are not as obvious in your documentation. You may be right... But others need to understand *the reasoning* for your decision.

What evidence do you have at the point you make a recommendation?

- *Assessment of needs:* This is the start of information-gathering, but remember that this is like an MOT – things can and will change between this and the home adaptation.

- *Observations:* These are key in evidencing your decision-making. Observations are compared with what you have read and heard, and either confirm what you have been told or lead you to more investigations. People will often have a clear idea of what they think they need and how best to achieve it. Your role is to take this on board and to then consider the information available and make recommendations appropriate to the situation. For example, they, or those supporting them, may believe a ground floor adaptation is needed. If you observe that they can negotiate stairs, then ground floor facilities are unlikely to be necessary or appropriate.

- *Information:* This is the information gathered from external sources such as medical reports. Confirmation of diagnosis, prognosis, planned surgery or rehabilitation – these all inform the decision-making process and your conclusions.

- *Knowledge:* We have separated knowledge and experience. Knowledge is structured information relating to adaptations, and experience is what you have learned through practice. Legislation and Building

Regulations are examples of knowledge-based evidence. You know that there are criteria and rules that can inform and constrain what you wish to achieve. Your knowledge and understanding of legislation, regulations, policies and guidance will enable you to make recommendations that are appropriate.

- *Experience:* Experiential learning provides a different type of knowledge. Adapting a property type informs your decision-making when you have a similar situation. You cannot write 'adaptations at x address demonstrated that y can be achieved'. Case notes can record this has been achieved at a similar type of property via a particular method, thus indicating that the identified outcome is feasible. Equally, noting that a similar property could not be adapted due to x or y assists with understanding why you have not suggested that as an option. Experience, and learning from it, is important, but remember that not every situation remains the same, and there may be new solutions that resolve the issue. So keep an open mind as others may have alternative options that will achieve the result you are aiming for.

Practical information-gathering

Assessment, **activity (or task) analysis** and **models of practice/theoretical frameworks** underpin your practice and have relevance to your decision-making. A cyclical assessment process forms part of the professional reasoning cycle. Within this, or as a specific information-gathering tool, is activity or task analysis. This key occupational therapy tool can be overlooked as you move from novice to experienced practitioner. Where someone you are supporting indicates or demonstrates a particular difficulty, going back to basics is a good way of unpicking a situation. Here we use the sequential unpacking of an activity, but we also draw on models and theoretical frameworks. To illustrate:

Difficulty getting in and out of the bath due to an orthopaedic condition?
The biomechanical model will identify affected movement patterns.

A child not achieving independence in personal care?
The developmental model will indicate if this is an appropriate activity at that age and stage.

If you are considering recommendations that promote positive risk-taking or that have restrictive elements, it is essential to summarize these in a risk evaluation report (see the Appendix). You need to evidence professional reasoning, demonstrating why a particular course of action was taken or not pursued. Having this information readily available saves time and effort for those who follow – because the allocated practitioner has changed or the casework has been reopened for a review or a new intervention.

We are not saying that case notes and reports should be full of academic references. Your knowledge combines with experience to provide the foundations of your practice. If challenged, you should be able to justify your recommendations through well-reasoned thought processes.

Being a reflective practitioner

As a reflective practitioner aware of your biases or preconceptions, your response should ensure that the needs of the person are reflected in your interventions. It can be an uncomfortable process, considering yourself in this way, but we all have unconscious biases resulting from life experiences, knowledge and areas in which we lack experience. You are likely aware of the biases some hold in relation to ethnicity, belief and culture, but there are many other ways in which you respond to people or situations that result from preconceptions. These may include aspects relating to 'bad habits' such as smoking, or drug taking, or relate to age or disability.

The role of supervision and peer support in professional reasoning

As you start in your role assessing for and recommending housing adaptations, the support you receive from colleagues is invaluable and remains relevant as you progress. Discussions that enable you to reflect and re-evaluate are key to ensuring that your recommendations remain relevant, and any changing circumstances are considered. (In independent practice, we highly recommend linking with a peer support group or with a supervisor.)

What do you want from a supervisor? While having someone with all the answers in their back pocket (or indeed, a copy of this book) is useful, it does not support development. A coaching approach to supervision or mentoring will enable and encourage you to understand the process by which you evaluate situations and reach conclusions.

'Why...?' is a good question in many situations, but within supervision you will need more. Guided questions that will support you and help develop discussion include:

- What alternatives have you identified?

- How will that affect others in the household?

- Is this achievable in the space available?

- Are there any interim solutions to the identified need?

It may be that you develop a list that you apply to situations yourself, but the process of discussion and enquiry can be invaluable in guiding your decision-making.

This chapter has discussed the importance of professional reasoning and the role it plays in communicating your findings and the reasons behind your interventions. It offers an understanding of what considered professional reasoning brings to your practice. The clinical reasoning cycle (Levett-Jones *et al.* 2010) is used to support this understanding, and offers a framework to support practice. Housing adaptations require complex decision-making with major long-term implications (Clutton *et al.* 2006). Therefore the key to achieving successful outcomes is in evidencing, understanding and articulating your thought processes.

6

Legislation and Guidance for the Provision of Housing Adaptations in the United Kingdom

SHANE ELLIOTT, DAVID OWEN,
JILL PRITCHARD AND KATE SHEEHAN

Knowledge check

* What part of the UK do you practice in?

* Do you know what legislation and guidance is used in your part of the UK?

* Can you list some categories of adaptations that are eligible for funding in your part of the UK?

As you most probably know, housing is a devolved matter for Northern Ireland, Scotland and Wales, and in England is still under the control of the UK Government. There are differences between each of the UK home nations on the level of funding, types of facilities provided and the financial impacts on individuals.

This chapter aims to give you an overview of what legislation is in place for each of the home nations. The contents of this chapter have been written by occupational therapists who are practising in the social care and housing field, and by no means constitutes legal advice. We would always advocate that you familiarize yourself with the legislation and policy in the nation where you practice, and the adaptations policy for the housing authority you refer to.

England
What are the funding routes for adaptations?
The primary funding for home adaptations is the Disabled Facilities Grant (DFG), which is available to all individuals regardless of their housing **tenure**. Tenants in local authorities tend to source their funding via the local authority revenue budgets and do not need to apply for a DFG; the authority is responsible for funding any identified adaptations.

England differs from Wales and Northern Ireland in that there is a wider range of local government structures and the maximum mandatory DFG is currently set at £30,000.

The English local authorities have a range of differing structures:

- County councils, with responsibility for social care assessments, and district councils, which are responsible for administering DFGs, via their housing responsibilities; an example is Lincolnshire County Council.

- Unitary authorities, which have responsibility for social care assessments and for administering DFGs; examples are Bristol City Council and the London Boroughs.

- City regions, which are responsible for certain aspects of housing policy, but not the administration of the DFG.

The legislation listed in Table 3 is the basis for adaptation funding in England.

Table 3. Legislation in England

Legislation	What it does
Housing Grants, Construction and Regeneration Act 1996	• Section 23 sets out what facilities can be funded by a DFG.
The Regulatory Reform (Housing Assistance) (England and Wales) Order 2002	• The Order allows local authorities to develop a range of options to use DFG funding, provided these options are in a published policy.

The Disabled Facilities Grants (Maximum Amounts and Additional Purposes) (England) Order 2008	• Section 2 increased the maximum grant amount to £30,000. • Section 3 added access to the garden, balcony or yard that belongs to the dwelling being considered for grant funding and adjoining land for a houseboat.
Chronically Sick and Disabled Persons Act 1970	• Section 2 requires local authorities to provide a range of services to eligible residents including home adaptations, 'designed to secure his [sic] greater safety, comfort or convenience'. The Act did not state to what extent or level. • Only relevant to children under 19 years of age. • The Act has been repealed for adults as there are provisions within the Care Act 2014 for providing adaptations.
Children Act 1989	• Section 17 of the Act confirms that a child is 'in need' if he or she is disabled, and the local authority provides for assistance for children in need, which includes disabled children. This could include the funding of essential equipment and adaptations. • Schedule 2 outlines the range of services that can be provided. Paragraph 6 of this Schedule requires that local authorities provide services to minimize the effect on disabled children of their disabilities, and gives such children the opportunity to lead lives that are as normal as possible.

Care Act 2014	• Section 1 of the Act states that there is a general duty to promote the wellbeing of that individual.
	• Wellbeing is defined to include nine components with 1, 4 and 8 being pertinent to adaptations:
	  – Personal dignity
	  – Control by the individual over day-to-day life (including over care and support, or support, provided to the individual and the way in which it is provided)
	  – Suitability of living accommodation.
	• Funding is available for minor adaptations up to £1,000, free of charge.

Housing Grants, Construction and Regeneration Act 1996

Where the DFG is being applied for on behalf of a person under 18 years, there is no means test. Where the applicant is over the age of 18, they are required to undertake a means test, and this will determine if the applicant must contribute towards the grant.

Those in receipt of certain means-tested benefits may be exempt from means testing and can be 'passported' through this process. This applies to those who own their own property, rent from a private landlord or from a housing association, or a tenant of a stock transfer housing association.

There is a caveat with housing association-owned properties: the tenant is expected to fund their assessed contribution. Some housing associations have agreements where they also contribute to the DFG, which is negotiated between the local authority and the relevant housing association, and is by no means universal or uniform across England.

Council tenants are generally not subject to a means test as any adaptations required in this tenure are usually funded from the housing revenue account. There is an understanding that any applicant will live in the property for five years. Some local authorities may place a land charge on the property; this is more common in circumstances where funding has exceeded the statutory requirement or discretionary funding has been used to enable the works to go ahead.

The categories of adaptations that can generally be funded via the DFG are set out in Section 23 of the Act. These are outlined in Chapter 7.

The role of the occupational therapist is usually to assess what is 'necessary and appropriate' to meet the person's needs, for example, if it is necessary to provide access to a bathroom, the appropriate solution could be a **stairlift** or a **through floor lift** to access existing facilities or extend the property. The specific recommendation would be justified by a therapist's clear professional reasoning documentation.

The Regulatory Reform (Housing Assistance) (England and Wales) Order 2002

The Order provides general and more flexible powers for local housing authorities to provide assistance for housing renewal, including home adaptations. Local authorities have to comply with the following to make use of the **regulatory reform order** (RRO):

- There must be a formally adopted policy in place; this will indicate how they will use the RRO powers to meet the needs of its residents.

- The policy must be published within the local community, and a copy of the full policy should be publicly available, at no cost.

- A summary document must be available on request.

The general power under Article 3 of this Order enables local authorities to give discretionary assistance for minor adaptations to fulfil needs not covered by mandatory DFGs, by avoiding the procedural complexities of mandatory DFGs. The aim should be to deliver a much quicker remedy for urgent adaptations. There is no restriction on the amount of assistance that can be given.

An example of its use is introducing no means test for the first £5000 of works. This has enabled smaller works to be completed quickly, such as stairlifts, shower adaptations and external ramps. Another example is providing a top-up for works that exceed the mandatory maximum grant, where the applicant cannot find additional funding to allow the necessary works to be completed.

Chronically Sick and Disabled Persons Act 1970

Provision for assessing the needs of people with disabilities is contained in the Act. The provisions are wide-ranging and include an assessment for adaptations to the home. This Acts places a duty on local authorities to fund adaptations that are designed to 'secure his [sic] greater safety, comfort or convenience'. The Act only applies to children under the age of 19.

Local authorities can use this Act to provide top-ups for grants (which can be means tested), although legally a local authority can restrict provision due to resources. Children's Services have a responsibility for ensuring that assessments of needs that might best be met by the provision of equipment and/or adaptations are carried out under the Act.

Children Act 1989

The Act states that authorities must provide a range of family support services for children in need; the definition of 'children in need' includes disabled children.

Schedule 2 to the Act requires that local authorities provide services to minimize the effect on disabled children of their disabilities, and give such children the opportunity to lead lives that are as normal as possible.

Section 17 imposes a duty on local authorities to safeguard and promote the welfare of children in their area who are in need by providing a range and level of services appropriate to the child's needs.

Section 23 imposes a duty on the local authority to provide accommodation for a child in local authority care and to maintain that child. If the child is disabled, it is their duty to ensure accommodation is suitable for that child.

Care Act 2014

The Act aims to ensure the wellbeing of people at the centre of the assessment, process and care provision.

The Act places a duty on a local authority to carry out care and support functions that promote integration, including housing, and to provide or arrange services that remove, delay or reduce the need for care.

There is a legal duty to cooperate with external partners including **housing providers**, and the Act promotes the pooling of resources between health, housing and social care services.

There should be funding available up to £1000 for minor adaptations (and equipment), and this must be free of charge.

Wales
How are adaptations considered?
The Social Services and Wellbeing (Wales) Act 2014 (SSWBA) places a duty on a local authority to assess an individual (adult, child or carer) where they appear to have care and support needs. The SSWBA applies equally to adults and children.

Section 3 of the Act deals with the assessment of need, and some of the following areas must be addressed: it focuses on supporting individuals to carry out self-care and domestic routines; having suitable living accommodation and access to work, learning and leisure opportunities; and maintaining and developing family and other significant relationships.

Section 4 of the Act deals with provision of care and support, although it is silent on the provision of adaptations. Guidance from the Association for Directors of Social Services Cymru suggested that DFG funding can be used to achieve some of the wellbeing outcomes defined by the SSWBA, and should be considered as part of a preventive approach to care and support planning. The guidance states that meeting the objectives of the SSWBA is a corporate responsibility, and not just that of social care departments.

Typically an occupational therapist will assess an individual and will offer an opinion on the needs of the individual and will define what adaptations are necessary and appropriate, and communicate these needs to the housing authority. The final decision on what will be provided rests with the housing authority or Welsh Government in respect to housing associations.

What are the funding routes for adaptations?
The primary means of funding in adaptations in Wales is the DFG and it is operated in a similar way as in England, although there are some differences. In Wales DFG funding is available to individuals who own their own home, rent from a private landlord or are a tenant of a stock transfer housing association (former local authority-owned properties).

Where the individual rents their home from the local authority (council tenant), the authority must fund the adaptation.

The other means of funding adaptations is a Physical Adaptation Grant (PAG). This is available to tenants of housing associations that have been set up as independent entities, and since April 2022 stock transfer housing associations can also apply for a PAG; this funding is not available to tenants of local authority-owned properties.

Disabled Facilities Grant (DFG)

The legislation in Table 4 is the basis for DFG funding in Wales.

Table 4. Legislation in Wales

Legislation	What it does
Housing Grants, Construction and Regeneration Act 1996	• Section 23 sets out what facilities can be funded by a DFG.
The Regulatory Reform (Housing Assistance) (England and Wales) Order 2002	• The Order allows local authorities to develop a range of options to use DFG funding, provided these options are in a published policy.
The Disabled Facilities Grants (Maximum Amounts and Additional Purposes) (Wales) Order 2008	• Section 2 increased the maximum DFG to £36,000. • Section 3 added access to the garden, balcony or yard that belongs to the dwelling being considered for grant funding and adjoining land for a houseboat.

In Wales a person under the age of 18 does not have to contribute towards a DFG. Persons over the age of 18 are still subject to a means test for large-scale works, and the means test has been removed for small- and medium-type works, as described in Table 6.

The categories of adaptations that can generally be funded by the DFG are set out in Section 23 of the Act and are discussed in Chapter 7.

There is one caveat to the DFG: some Welsh local authorities will fund ceiling tracked hoists via the DFG and others are funded by social care directly, and maintain ownership and responsibility for maintenance and repair.

Physical Adaptation Grant (PAG)

The Welsh Government says that to be eligible for this grant the applicant must be a tenant of a housing association, be disabled or be an older person. The Welsh Government (2022, p.4) states that PAGs should be used for the same purpose as DFGs, as laid out in Section 23 of the 1996 Act.

Generally, an occupational therapist is required to assess the individual and make recommendations to the housing association. The housing association itself then decides on the best solution and will apply to the Welsh Government for funding before works start; once works are completed the housing association will be reimbursed.

The Welsh Government provides a list of the areas that can be funded (see Table 5).

Table 5. Adaptation categories

Areas	Examples
Bathroom adaptations	Level-access shower, wash and dry toilet, body dryers etc.
Lifts	Stairlifts, through floor lifts etc.
Hoists	Ceiling tracked hoists etc.
Kitchen adaptations	Height-adjustable work surfaces etc.
Access	Ramps, alteration to doorways, alterations to pathways etc.
Other	Door opening systems, door restrictors etc.

The Welsh Government (2022, p.6) guidance further states that PAGs may not be used for some of the following purposes:

- Making the property larger or other alterations to relieve overcrowding

- Adaptations to communal areas, except where this is needed to allow the resident to access their home

- Landscaping or levelling of gardens, patios and other areas, except where this is needed to allow the resident primary access to their home.

Notionally, while there isn't a specified maximum amount that a PAG can fund, it is generally accepted that the maximum funding available is £36,000, which is in line with the DFG.

Adaptation standards in Wales

The Welsh Government has established minimum standards that define timescales for assessment and delivery, who should be involved in prescribing an adaptation and categories for adaptations (Welsh Government 2019).

Adaptations have been split into small, medium and large, and each category has a general description of types of works and who should be involved in prescribing them, and how long it should take, from assessment to installation of the works. Table 6 breaks this down further.

Table 6. Adaptation service standards

	Small	Medium	Large
Definition	Not a specialist solution, no building or planning approval needed, e.g., grab rails, key safe, mopstick handrail etc.	Major home modification, but planning/building approval not needed, e.g., bathroom adaptations, stairlift etc. or combination thereof.	Structural alteration needed. Planning/building approval needed, specialist or innovative solutions needed, e.g., through floor lift, property extension, relocation of bathroom etc.
Time frame for assessment	No assessment required.	Within 2 months from first contact with provider to being assessed by a competent person. When recommendation is determined to be needed, the written report completed within 2 weeks of the decision.	Within 2 months from first contact with provider to being assessed by a competent person. When recommendation is determined to be needed, the written report completed within 2 weeks of the decision.
Time frame for installation of solution	Within 3 weeks if urgent or 4 weeks if routine recommendation being made.	Within 4 months from the date of recommendation.	Within 15 months of recommendation.
Who should prescribe	Assessment may be needed from a trusted assessor.	Occupational therapist or trusted assessor.	Occupational therapist.

Northern Ireland
What are the funding routes for adaptations?
There is an interdepartmental approach to funding adaptation provision in Northern Ireland, with collaboration between the Department of Health and Department for Communities through the Interdepartmental Adaptations Programme Board. This Board sets the policy and strategic direction for the delivery of adaptations.

Health and Social Care (HSC) Trusts, via occupational therapy services, are responsible for carrying out assessments of need to identify adaptations deemed to be necessary and appropriate. Following assessment and having established a need, provision is made in collaboration with the Northern Ireland Housing Executive (NIHE), which administers the appropriate funding and will determine if the work is reasonable and practicable.

Decisions regarding need are made in line with regionally agreed best practice guidance and the processes outlined in the *Interdepartmental Housing Adaptations Design Toolkit* (Department for Communities 2022).

Funding routes for adaptations are dependent on tenure, as outlined in Table 7.

Table 7. Funding routes

Tenure	Funding route
Private sector: owner-occupier/ private rental	HSC Trusts provide a range of minor works in the private sector including grab rails, stair rails and home lifts.
	The DFG is available for major adaptation provision in the private sector for owner-occupiers and private landlords. The DFG is a means-tested process administered by the NIHE and funded by the Department for Communities. Means testing does not apply to under-18s.
	Eligible works are outlined in Section 54 of the Housing (Northern Ireland) Order 2003.
Social sector: NIHE stock	The NIHE funds both minor and major adaptations in full for their own stock. A range of minor works that do not require occupational therapy assessment is included in the Interdepartmental Housing Adaptations Design Toolkit.
Social sector: Housing association stock	Housing associations fund major adaptations via the Disability Adaptation Grant (DAG), administered by the Development Programme Group in the NIHE in line with the Adaptations Guide.[1]
	As for NIHE stock, a range of minor works can be provided by the housing associations without the need for occupational therapy assessment.

Current adaptation standards

Adaptations are built in accordance with the *Interdepartmental Housing Adaptations Design Toolkit* (Department for Communities 2022), which includes a matrix of space standards for the most frequently requested rooms, for example, the toilet, shower room and bedrooms. The matrix includes three

---

1   www.communities-ni.gov.uk/adaptations-guide

levels of space standards, determined by complexity and reflecting the level of an individual's function, ranging from the ambulant person to the assisted wheelchair user. Table 8 outlines the standards for different tenures.

Table 8. Adaptation standards

New-build: social sector	New-build general needs social housing is currently built to Lifetime Home standards (currently under review), and focuses on access and future adaptability. This is complemented by a target of 10% of new-builds to be built to wheelchair-accessible standards.[2]
New-build: private sector	Private sector properties are built in accordance with the Building Regulations outlined in Section 7 of *Access to and Use of Buildings. Technical Booklet R. Building Regulations Guidance* (Department of Finance and Personnel 2012). The Building Regulations focus primarily on visitability to the property, including external access, horizontal/vertical circulation, access to a toilet and heights of switches/sockets. They do not address or provide for full wheelchair accessibility within the property.

Primary legislation

Primary legislation exists in both housing and health, which underpin adaptation provision. These are listed in Table 9.

Table 9. Legislation in Northern Ireland

Legislation	What it does
The Housing (Northern Ireland) Order 2003	• Sections 50–55 set out the legislation in relation to the DFG.
Health and Personal Social Services (Northern Ireland) Order 1972	• This enabling legislation creates powers to provide welfare services to people in need. Health and Social Care Trusts have a duty 'to provide or secure the provision of personal social services in Northern Ireland designed to promote the social welfare of the people of Northern Ireland'. • Article 2 defines a 'person in need'. • Article 15 refers to making arrangements for advice and provision of facilities, including accommodation.

cont.

---

2   www.communities-ni.gov.uk/wheelchair-housing

Legislation	What it does
Chronically Sick and Disabled Persons (Northern Ireland) Act 1978	• Section 1: Identify numbers and identities of disabled people and ensure service information. • Section 2(e): Provide assistance to disabled people in arranging for the carrying out of any works of adaptation in his [sic] home or the provision of any additional facilities designed to secure his greater safety, comfort or convenience. • Section 3: Duties of the Housing Executive: when considering the needs of any district with respect to the provision of further housing accommodation shall have regard to the special needs of chronically sick and disabled persons; and any proposals for the provision of new housing shall distinguish any houses which the Executive proposes to provide which make special provision for the needs of those persons.
Disabled Persons (Northern Ireland) Act 1989	• Section 3: Disabled person or authorized representatives to make representation regarding assessment for or provision of services. • Section 8 takes into account abilities of carers where care is substantial and informal.
The Health and Social Care Trusts (Establishment) (Amendment) Order (Northern Ireland) 2022	This legislation came into operation in April 2022 and resulted in the dissolution of certain functions from the Department of Health to the Health and Social Care Trusts. These functions include duties outlined as above in the: • Health and Personal Social Services (Northern Ireland) Order 1972 • Chronically Sick and Disabled Persons (Northern Ireland) Act 1978 • Disabled Persons (Northern Ireland) Act 1989.

Scotland
What are the funding routes for adaptations?
The way that 'major' adaptations are funded in Scotland is directly related to housing tenure and differs across owner-occupiers and private tenants, local authority tenants and housing association tenants (see Table 10).

Table 10. Funding routes

Tenure	Permission required	Funding	Works
Owner-occupier	No	Can be covered by a local authority mandatory grant if the work is considered essential. Grants are made either at 80% or 100% if the person receives certain benefits. Any remaining costs must be met by the homeowner. The local authority has discretionary powers to top up the grant.	The work must be organized by the homeowner but this can be supported by the local authority or organizations such as Care and Repair. However, work should not commence before written approval of a grant is received. Any relevant planning permissions should also have been received.
Private tenant	Yes	Can be covered by a local authority mandatory grant if the work is considered essential. Grants are made either at 80% or 100% if the person receives certain benefits. Any remaining costs must be met by the tenant.	The work ought to be organized by the tenant, with the agreement of the landlord. However, work should not commence before written approval of a grant is received. Any relevant planning permissions should also have been received.
Local authority tenant	Yes	The work will be paid for in full by the local authority (subject to availability of funding).	The local authority will organize any works.
Housing association tenant	Yes	The work will be paid for by the housing association, subject to availability of funding.	The housing association will organize any works.

'Minor' adaptations are usually funded by the local authority social care service.

Assessment
In most situations and across all tenures, the assessment of need will be carried out by an occupational therapist; however, all partners are encouraged to put self-assessment and 'fast track'-type arrangements in place for straightforward cases to avoid unnecessary delays.

Eligibility

Each local authority and health and social care partnership will have its own eligibility criteria and prioritization approach, which will be published on their websites. Table 11 summarizes Scottish legislation in this area of practice.

Table 11. Legislation in Scotland

Legislation	What it does
Housing Scotland Act 2006	• Requires local authorities to provide assistance to homeowners when adaptations are required to make the property suitable for a disabled person (or to reinstate a property that has already been adapted). The provisions of the 2006 Act do not cover adaptations to mobile homes.
Implementing the Housing (Scotland) Act 2006	• Parts 1 and 2: Statutory Guidance for Local Authorities: Volume 6, Work to Meet the Needs of Disabled People, published in 2009 ('the 2009 guidance').
	• The 2006 Act (Section 72) also requires local authorities to publish a statement of the criteria by which it decides whether to provide assistance and in what form. This is known as a 'Statement of Assistance'. However, the 2006 Act does state that any works undertaken to provide 'standard amenities', i.e., a toilet, sink or shower, must be assisted by a grant (known as a mandatory grant). This reflects a pre-existing duty authorities had under the Housing (Scotland) Act 1987 regarding standard amenities.
Housing (Scotland) Act 2006 (Scheme of Assistance) Regulations 2008	• State that where the adaptations required are essential to the disabled person's needs and the required work is structural (or involves permanent changes to the house), the applicant must also be awarded a mandatory grant.
	• They do not specify any particular types of works that ought to be deemed eligible for a mandatory grant. Therefore, each local authority determines what it considers to be a structural (i.e., major) adaptation.
	• If any required adaptations identified do not qualify for financial assistance, the 2008 Regulations (Section 3) state that the local authority must provide advice and information to help the applicant to fund the adaptations required.
Relevant Adjustments to Common Parts (Disabled Persons) (Scotland) Regulations 2020	• These mean that a disabled homeowner or tenant can request adaptations to the communal areas of their buildings provided a majority of the other homeowners agree. A tenant (with the landlord's consent) or homeowner can, with the agreement of the *majority* of their homeowners, install a ramp or other adaptation within communal areas of a building. This will make buildings, such as blocks of flats or tenements, more accessible for disabled people.

Chronically Sick and Disabled Persons Act 1970	• Places a duty on local authorities to provide support when it has been identified that a disabled person has certain needs, including the need for assistance in carrying out works of adaptation in their home, regardless of tenure.

Integration authorities

As part of the integration of health and social care, the duties local authorities currently have in relation to certain aspects of housing support, including equipment and adaptations, have been delegated to Integration Authorities (under the Public Bodies (Joint Working) (Scotland) Act 2014. This includes functions under the Housing Act 2001 in regard to assistance for housing purposes (Section 92) and under the Housing Scotland Act 2006 relating to the adaptation of a house for a disabled person to make it suitable for the accommodation, welfare or employment of that person (Section 71(1)(b)) (Scottish Government 2015).

In effect, this means that:

- The duty to assess for an adaptation has been delegated to Integration Authorities.

- The planning for and resources to undertake adaptations have been delegated to Integration Authorities.

- The resource to fund housing adaptations – including for local authority tenants – has passed to Integration Authorities.

- Integration Authorities have powers and associated budgets delegated for the planning and delivery of advice and assistance to housing associations/registered social landlords in relation to adaptations (although local authorities have rarely used this provision).

The delegation of responsibility for housing adaptations to Integration Authorities does not alter the duties outlined under the 2006 Act or 2008 Regulations, for example the provision of mandatory grants or advice to those ineligible to a grant. In addition, although responsibility will lie with the Integration Authorities, delivery arrangements for adaptations will still be determined locally, although Integration Authorities will need to make sure that their obligation, under the Public Bodies Act, to take a person-centred approach is met (Scottish Government 2015).

Importantly, in the Scottish Government Advice Note[3] on the delegation of housing-related functions to the Integrated Authorities, including adaptations, the definition of an 'aid or adaptation' is as follows:

> An 'aid or adaptation' means any alteration or addition to the structure, access, layout or fixtures of accommodation, and any equipment or fittings installed or provided for use in accommodation, for the purpose of allowing a person to occupy, or to continue to occupy, the accommodation as their sole or main residence...

This therefore enables a person-centred approach to assessment of need in the widest sense.

Good practice in adaptations

While there are no nationally agreed standards for adaptations across Scotland, good practice guidance is provided via the Scottish Government.[4]

The Scottish Government has completed a review to streamline and accelerate the adaptations system, taking action to reduce the time it takes to apply for and receive support and maximizing the available resources. This developed recommendations improving the system so that it is fit and capable of dealing with the increased demand driven by an ageing population (Scottish Government 2021).

Other legislation, regulations and conventions
Equalities Act 2010

The Equalities Act updates the definition of disability from the previous one in the National Assistance Act 1948.

A person has a disability for the purposes of the Act if he or she has a physical or mental impairment, and the impairment has a substantial and long-term adverse effect on his or her ability to carry out normal day-to-day activities.

The document *Disability: Equality Act 2010* (Government Equalities Office 2013) further clarified what impairments could be included in the definition of a disability. Section A, paragraph A5 provides a list of impairments that could lead to a disability, including impairments with fluctuating and recurring effects (such as rheumatoid arthritis, fibromyalgia etc.), progressive

---

3   www.gov.scot/binaries/content/documents/govscot/publications/advice-and-guidance/2015/09/housing-advice-note/documents/00484861-pdf/00484861-pdf/govscot%3Adocument/00484861.pdf
4   www.gov.scot/publications/guidance-provision-equipment-adaptations-2

conditions (such as motor neurone disease etc.) and developmental conditions (such as autism spectrum disorder).

The Equalities Act applies to England, Wales and Scotland. The situation in Northern Ireland is somewhat different as this is a devolved matter with generally equal protections provided in a range of different statutes.[5]

Human Rights Act 1998

The Human Rights Act enables a person to defend their rights in UK courts, and compels public organizations (including central and devolved governments, the police and local authorities) to treat everyone equally, with fairness, dignity and respect.

The key areas relating to disabled people are:

- Right to life.

- Respect for privacy and family life.

- Freedom from discrimination.

The Act applies equally in all UK nations.

Health and Safety at Work Act 1974

This Act is the primary piece of legislation covering occupational health and safety in Great Britain. As occupational therapists we must understand that when recommending adaptations, they are not only to a client's home but also to a work environment for carers or personal assistants.

The Act sets out the general duties that:

- Employers have towards employees and members of the public.

- Employees have to themselves and to each other.

- Certain self-employed people have towards themselves and others.

The Act applies to England, Wales and Scotland. In Northern Ireland similar provisions have been made in the Health and Safety at Work (Northern Ireland) Order 1978.

The Manual Handling Operations Regulations 1992

These Regulations impose duties on employers and employees around safe moving and handling of people:

---

5   More information on the anti-discrimination protections in Northern Ireland can be found at: www.nidirect.gov.uk/articles/diversity-and-discrimination

- Where possible, avoid manual handling.

- If avoidance is not possible, assess the situation.

- Reduce the risks to the lowest level possible and practicable.

- Review the situation regularly.

When designing adaptations, a therapist must complete a risk assessment where moving and handling tasks are involved.

The Regulations apply to England, Wales and Scotland. In Northern Ireland similar provisions have been made in the Manual Handling Operations Regulations (Northern Ireland) 1992.

United Nations Convention on the Rights of Children 1989

- *Article 31* (Leisure, play and culture): play is recognized as a fundamental human right and children have the right to relax and play, and to join in a wide range of cultural, artistic and other recreational activities.

- *Article 23* (Children with disabilities): children who have any kind of disability have the right to special care and support, as well as all the rights in the Convention, so that they can live full and independent lives.

United Nations Convention on the Rights of Persons with Disabilities

The Convention sets out a range of protections that should be extended to those living with a disability. Many of the protections have been implemented in the range of health, social care and anti-discrimination legislation across all UK nations.

Conclusion

This has been a whistle-stop tour of the framework that supports the provision of adaptations in each of the UK nations. We can see that each nation has taken differing approaches to achieving the goal of ensuring that the home supports occupational engagement by reducing environmental barriers and facilitating choice and control.

The system is by no means perfect, and it has many flaws, particularly on its bias towards physical disability; however, the system we have is better than nothing at all. Legislation is always slow to move and keep up with the changes in the way we live as well as advances in healthcare and the treatment of disease and ill health.

As mentioned at the beginning, this chapter was written by occupational therapists, and not lawyers. As responsible practitioners who advocate for the people we work with, understanding the mechanisms that support our interventions is key, as it informs our practice, enables us to set realistic expectations and know what is likely to be funded. Knowing this supports our professional reasoning and enables us to be better advocates for the people we work with, and how far we may be able to flex the rules!

7

Occupational Therapy Key Skills

You have been given a case where the referral indicates a need for housing adaptations. What do you do next? Do you assess with a presumption that this is what is needed? Definitely not! There is a process you will need to go through before you get to the point of making a recommendation, even if the request was made by an occupational therapist or a member of the housing team.

We describe occupational therapists working in social care or housing as the multi-tool of our profession. Occupational therapists are 'specialist-generalists'. You may think this sounds like an oxymoron, but you will require a detailed knowledge of a wide range of specialisms, from building solutions to equipment to moving and handling, and apply these to individual circumstances. All in all, an impressive skill set!

So where do we start?

Pre-visit steps

With information-gathering, you are quite the detective at this point in the process. You have many sources of information you can access before you even leave your workplace.

First, unpick information in the referral. This provides the person's name (always useful), age, address, family make-up and diagnosis or disability as well as reasons for the referral. You may learn of other professionals involved, and previous involvements with your service and future plans, such as surgery.

Having reviewed the referral, revisit any notes or information from previous involvements by your team. This can be supplemented by discussions with those completing that work – but a word of warning, do not let this colour your view at this time. You will be completing your own assessment and observations before reaching any conclusions.

Next, you yourself are a resource. Do you know the person, the area or the type of dwelling? Your knowledge is part of building a picture of the person's situation (but again, this must not mean that you make presumptions before your assessment).

Once you have got to this point there is still more to discover. Depending on the permissions given you may be able to contact involved professionals (if permission isn't in place, then you can get verbal consent when you first make contact with the person).

Who would you want to speak with or contact at this point? Physiotherapists will be able to advise on mobility, current interventions and intended outcomes. This is useful if the request is for a stairlift and the person is working to achieve independence on stairs. Information from consultants can provide the prognosis, the impact of treatment programmes and contraindications. Other occupational therapists will provide a range of information, and for children, understanding their presentation at school can be illuminating.

Next, head to the internet – not cyber-stalking, but utilizing open-source information.

Online maps are amazing – so much information. But don't forget to check when the image was taken, as not all are refreshed on the same schedule. Starting with a map – where is the property situated? What is the area around it like (garden, public space, neighbouring properties)? A satellite view offers more context than a map, and then there is also street view – such a handy resource. This will help you identify exactly which property you will be visiting (and parking options, if needed). Once you have identified the property you can get an idea of what type of building it is and its construction – not 100% reliable, as looks can be deceiving, but it's a start.

You can take an image (screenshot or snip) and save it to a file if you think that it will be useful, as this will save time later when you want to check details.

The ability to measure distance from a satellite view is useful but not fully accurate. Is there mention of a need for off-road parking in the referral? Does the property appear close to the road or pavement? It supports understanding what is achievable before you have even left the office.

A handy hint for properties that are off the beaten path or not easily located – use what3words.[1] This divides the world into 3m squares, each identified by a unique combination of three words.

Street view is the gift that keeps giving, as not only can we learn about the property and garden, but also the surrounding area. Is the property on a corner or a junction? Is there a dropped kerb? Is there any street furniture in the vicinity? (Why should a post box or lamp post etc. matter? If there is a need for off-road parking these could affect the ability to create this.) Bus stops, tube or rail links are key for accessing the person's community. Looking at neighbouring properties helps with understanding what is feasible. If an extension is needed, do other properties have them, and if so, where are they located? A request for a hardstanding – are there precedents set on neighbouring properties? (Although again, check the date.)

Planning portals allow you to view planning applications. This gives access to information on previous works completed at that address. It may indicate that there is no scope for additional development, or if a request was declined and the reason. Another useful aspect of planning portal access is the ability to track progress of planning applications, highlighting the next stage of your involvement. The portals are easy to navigate and searchable by postcode. Once you have identified the relevant record, note the reference number, as this will speed up access later.

A bit left-field for some, but previous property listings often have images and floor plans included. Historic listings add details that will assist in your understanding of a building, although the room sizes are listed as guidance, and subsequent changes may have been made to the layout.

Finally, you can arrange an appointment to complete a home visit. This is another opportunity to gather information. Does the person work or attend school? Would they prefer a family member to be present? Do they ask you to be careful where you park, as there are tensions with neighbours…?

If you haven't got consent on record to contact other professionals, this is a good time to request this and record it as part of your call. (If the policy is to have written consent, you can take the relevant form with you on your visit.) Images are useful for giving context in later discussions and as an aide-mémoire. Also, you can gain prior consent for taking photographs during your visit, although reassurance that images will be stored appropriately should always be given.

---

1   https://what3words.com/pretty.needed.chill

On consent to contact other professionals, it is worth mentioning that if it is not given, you are pretty much stymied. Your role in adaptations means that you must liaise with a wide range of people (see Chapter 4). If you do not have permission to gather information and understand the wider situation, it is appropriate to advise those you are supporting that your ability to address their needs will be limited by their decision.

This is an opportunity for you to confirm why you are visiting (what we think is expected is not always what the person thinks is happening), any changes in circumstances since the referral was made, and to confirm the address. This last one can be frustrating. You expect the information passed to you to be up to date, but this isn't always the case. Yes, your research is not as relevant, but it is a 'chicken and egg' situation as you may have conversations that don't fully make sense if you haven't made yourself familiar with the wider picture.

If your team's approach is to send out a letter with an appointment for the initial contact, then you'll be skipping this step, but, on the other hand, a quick call the day before the appointment to check if it's still okay can be useful.

This section has been written as if you are going out on your initial assessment visit, but this isn't always the case. You may have been working with someone for a while before the need for adaptation is identified. In this case, your approach will differ slightly, but it's always good to step back and take stock of a situation and to look at it with fresh eyes.

Your home visit toolkit

There is nothing more frustrating than turning up and realizing that you haven't got everything you need. We have all done it at some point, but having a 'home visit toolkit' can limit the times you find yourself with that sinking feeling:

- *Address and contact details:* Handy if you turn up and there is no one answering the door! Have you got the right property? Have they remembered your visit, or has something happened that has called them away? If they aren't in, having a 'Sorry I missed you' card is always useful, but nowadays a voicemail or text message evidences that you did attend as agreed.

- *Identification:* Useful if you are making notes or taking images outside a property, as neighbours may challenge you. So, beside the point that you should always have this with you, official identification enables you to reassure others you are not scoping out a property for nefarious reasons.

- *Something to write notes on:* Usually pen and paper, but if you have a tablet or laptop with a touchscreen, use this and save the file, making it accessible. If you use pen and paper, taking images of your notes/sketches and uploading these is useful. Neatness isn't important at this point; having the information to hand when you need it is.

- *A phone or camera:* Images aid recall but also assist discussion or demonstrate an issue. When trying to unpick a situation and look for solutions, you can have better outcomes if those you are discussing it with can visualize what you are describing. It goes without saying that you should not use your own device, and transfer images as soon as possible. See the Appendix for an example of an environmental assessment document.

- *Steel tape measure:* At a minimum this should be 5m, as this covers the size of most rooms in the UK.

- *'Soft' tape measure:* You may need to measure the person you are working with to understand areas of need. If someone has a very wide gait and there is a narrow doorway, you will need to understand the space required. Using a steel tape measure could be viewed as objectifying the person, while 'soft' tape measures are more personalized and appropriate.

An optional addition:

- *Digital tape measure:* These have become more affordable in recent years. The laser type is more accurate than the infrared option, which can struggle to accurately measure where there are reflective surfaces, such as in bathrooms and kitchens.

A note: This section is written from the perspective of an occupational therapist working in housing or social care, but has relevance for others completing **environmental assessments**.

The visit

We have focused on traditional dwellings, but if a boat, caravan or mobile home is a person's primary residence, legislation allows for this to be adapted.

Your assessment of the situation starts as you *approach the property*. How busy is the road? Parking locations? As you move towards the entrance, note aspects including:

- *Pathways:* Width, length, state of repair.

- *Steps:* Height, width, depth, number.

- *Ramps:* Width, length, platforms, rails, upstands.

- *Entrance points:* Location(s), type (shared, lobby areas), method of access (keypad, lock, intercom).

- *Stairs:* Open/enclosed, rails.

- *Lighting:* Type (street, perimeter, security), location, coverage.

This is where your camera is useful, but you may feel more comfortable taking images as you leave – just don't forget! Also, images taken from the pavement or road don't require specific permission but can be concerning for neighbours (see above). The 'Home access' video (1 minute 18 seconds) is available to download at https://library.jkp.com/redeem with the code EDKQQWA.

Now we start to get into specifics as you have rung the doorbell/used the intercom/knocked on the door:

- *How long does it take for the door to be answered?* This may indicate an area of need. Are they having difficulty negotiating access to that entrance due to mobility issues or fatigue? Or they may not have heard the bell or your knock the first time...

- *The person:* Your observations start as they invite you in and direct you to where they want you to be. You have the referral – did it mention mobility issues? What is their gait pattern? Do they use a walker or do they furniture walk? Any shortness of breath?

- *Access:* You will have noted steps already, but how easy are they for *you* to use? Your practical experience of them is part of your observation and experience of the environment. (It's not that you expect others to have the same experience, but you cannot discount yourself as part of your assessment toolkit.) As you move through the property, how wide are hallways and doors? You are not measuring these yet, but be aware of potential barriers and enablers.

Next you will be taking some time to discuss with the person their situation and understand what they consider to be the biggest barriers within their home. The room or space this takes place in may give you some clues to the person's preferred space to spend time in, but then again, if you haven't met them before, they may take you to a more 'formal' space. We have had initial conversations in kitchens, gardens, family rooms as well as in sitting rooms, which are clearly only used when guests visit.

How you gather information will vary. Your team may have a set list of questions or an information-gathering tool. This may allow for a general discussion or require you to follow a set format. Our preferred option is to ask the person to describe their day, starting from when they wake up and covering the full 24 hours, so we understand how well they sleep and how often they need to get up during the night (and why).

This conversational format allows them to explain the way they prefer to live and highlights key **occupations** and barriers they experience. We all have routines we follow; some people are more comfortable following these closely while others are flexible in their approach. Routines may be due to culture, upbringing, personality type and mental health issues or linked to medications or treatments. This initial conversation enables comparison of existing information, what they are telling you and clarification of household make-up.

If more than one person is present, you will gain an insight into relationships. Is one person providing all the information? Is this the person who has been referred to you, or is it their partner, parent, **caregiver** or child? Be mindful that in your information-gathering you ensure that the voice of the person you are supporting is heard. Others speaking for them is usually done to be helpful, but as a professional you must be aware that there are times when this should raise concern.

Once you have gained an understanding of how they live and their perceived barriers, identify the additional information you require. Generally, the next step will be to ask them to show you around their home. This provides you with two sources of information: your observation of the person and your observation of their environment. Combined with the information gathered this provides the basis on which you will formulate your interventions.

What are you going to ask them to demonstrate? This will vary and is down to your professional judgement. If they say they cannot get out of the bath, is it sensible to ask them to demonstrate this? A later visit with transfer equipment may be more appropriate as you really do not want to have to call for assistance with transfers. (If they insist on demonstrating that they can do it...and then get stuck, you will need to consider what are the suitable next actions. Sadly, this was learned the hard way!)

If they have difficulty rising from a seat that is a similar height as the toilet, it is a reasonable assumption that toilet transfers are problematic. Where someone has fatigue and/or shortness of breath, is it sensible to ask them to climb stairs if they only do this once a day? Consider the impact of your visit on their ability to function after you have left.

By the end of your visit, you will understand how that person lives their life...and how their home space is used. This means assessing the full layout of the property, including rooms that are infrequently used.

> A lesson learned: don't presume that just because someone lives alone that they are the only person at home! Working with someone who only climbed the stairs once a day due to shortness of breath and who had a ground floor bathroom, the issue was toileting overnight, so a review of the first floor room was agreed to identify if a toilet adaptation was an option. Door number one was her bedroom, numbers two and three were guest rooms. What she forgot to mention was her grandson was home from university and staying over for a couple of days. This was not the 9am wake-up call he was expecting!

In general, your understanding of the internal space will include:

- *Access:* Corridor, landing, door widths, steps, rails and bannisters.

- *Rooms:* Number, size, use, occupancy.

- *Utilities:* Type of heating – their ability to control this.

- *Upkeep:* This is not how tidy or clean the property is and if it meets 'your standards'; it is about the general state of the property – leaks, damp, draughts, heating, glazing, boiler type and age.

It is important that you understand the whole property, and not just the rooms that are used or what the person wants you to consider. If an adaptation is needed, always consider the use of existing space. It may be a challenge to suggest a sibling moves to a different bedroom (or they share a room when they have had their own space), that the youngest child doesn't necessarily have to have the smallest space, a play or craft room can be repurposed as a bedroom, or a guest room utilized in a different way. Consider all options. One space that may need to be 'protected' is a workspace if someone is employed and their work is home-based. It may need negotiation as to where this space is, but you cannot meet an area of need by removing employability and income. This may need unpicking as there has been a distinct move towards hybrid working since 2020. How this is interpreted in maintaining access to work/employment is evolving.

There are a number of areas you will consider to enable your understanding of the internal space, including:

- Your *notetaking*, including simple **sketch drawings** of key rooms to assist with recall and decision-making. During the visit these don't need to be neat and tidy, but just enough for you to recall key features.

- Using your *senses*: Your eyes will be working overtime to capture information, but they are not the only senses you will be using. Smell is key and shouldn't be ignored. Does the house smell musty, mouldy or of urine? Does it smell like the bin is overdue for emptying? Do these smells match up with what you are seeing?

- *Touch* is important as well. As you touch surfaces you can tell if they are going to offer support to the person. It's not about going around touching everything just in case; it's noting things that you experience during the assessment.

- *Proprioception* provides us with information about balance. If something makes you feel unbalanced, such as a sloping floor, uneven steps, loose flooring or rugs, others will experience the same. It may be they have learned to compensate for this, but you should be noting these potential hazards as part of your assessment.

- *Outside space:* Is an understanding of outside space important? Yes, definitely, as you do not want to restrict people so they can only manage inside but cannot access their outside space. Your assessment has already started as you walk towards the entrance to the property. Then you have your discussion with the person. Do they mention their outside space? If they don't, then ask them. Do they sit outside? Do they garden or do they hang their washing out to dry? Where are refuse bins stored and who puts them out? For children, do they play outdoors? If they don't, what prevents them? What level of supervision is required? You cannot enable access to all of the garden, but you can resolve certain issues.

So, you have now completed your information-gathering, what's next? You should be thanking those present for their time and patience – occupational therapists can ask some seemingly random questions and focus on aspects that may appear irrelevant... Summarize and agree what you will be focusing on. You cannot leave people with a sense of uncertainty – if you are unsure of your next actions, then say so, and that you will be discussing it with colleagues (line manager, peers, housing officer, etc.). If an assessment report is required before decisions are made, explain the next steps and likely timescales.

Although your focus is on the person and their physical space, you must also establish ownership, property tenure and residential status to identify the appropriate funding. You will need to know:

- *Ownership:* Owner-occupied, shared ownership, owned by a family member, landlord.

- *Rental status:* Privately rented, social housing (clarify if council stock or housing association).

- *Pattern of use:* Is this their main residence?

Post-visit actions

Then it's back to your workplace with (hopefully) sufficient time to reflect and start documenting your findings. This includes a clearer version of sketch drawings (if needed). We have included some resources (videos) to help you if you have not had experience in completing these.

Practical skills for measuring a room
We suggest you measure the room, but what does this mean? What is it that needs measuring and recording?

Measure at floor level – this identifies usable space. Measuring at waist height is easier, but consider a fireplace. At waist height its intrusion into a room is less than the size of the hearth below. You would be misled into thinking there was greater usable floor area. It is the same for a bulkhead over a set of stairs – there can be a significant difference in available space.

Measure the wall space and record the location of key fixed items. Furniture is moveable, but a window or door will determine how a space is used.

Videos are provided at https://library.jkp.com/redeem, which can be viewed using the code EDKQQA. First watch 'Measuring a room' (38 seconds), and then 'Creating a sketch drawing' (3 minutes 4 seconds).

Head to your bathroom and measure it, noting the key features and their location on a sketch drawing. Remember that gaps between items are as important as the items – this indicates available space to make changes or use equipment.

Assessment write-up

The assessment and information-gathering are complete and ready for synthesizing into a cohesive report. The presentation of this will differ depending on where you are in the occupational therapy process. It could be an initial assessment or an environmental assessment following a period of casework.

The beginning of any report must include:

- The name of the person being assessed (service user/patient/client).

- Their unique identifier (NHS no./case no. for social care).

- The assessor and their role.

- The address of the assessment location.

- The date and time of the assessment.

- Other people present.

You may be asked to complete an assessment of a property being considered for purchase or rent; think about how to describe this. Although the phrase 'property viewing' is commonly used, the process you will be completing is so much more – it is a thorough evaluation of suitability. 'Property viewing' implies you are just simply guiding someone around a building. The language you use is key to how your role is perceived. The evaluation you complete is complex, considering a wide range of factors, and your report is based on professional reasoning. Therefore, the phrase 'environmental assessment' and 'environmental assessment report' better reflects this complexity.

Soapbox moment over...

There are examples of initial assessment and environmental assessment forms in the Appendix, but it is most likely your team will already have a format in place.

The Person-Environment-Occupation-Performance (PEOP) model of practice (Baum *et al.* 2015) offers a structure you can use to organize the information you have gathered. To illustrate: saying that x has a strip wash rather than a bath or shower may be factually accurate but doesn't describe the whole picture. There is a significant difference in choosing to strip wash in the bathroom and lack of access forcing someone to strip wash in the kitchen.

It is good practice to add your drawings and images from the visit to the casework record to assist with future discussions and decision-making. Depending on the circumstances you may write up your summary and identify outcomes without further discussion, as you are clear in your analysis.

There will be times where you require support in unpicking a situation and applying professional reasoning. This may be due to the complexity of a situation (person, environment or occupation – or all three), or it may be because you lack knowledge. You cannot know everything and there is always a first-time experience. Seeking peer or manager support is not a failing or sign of weakness – more that you have reflected and recognized you need guidance – which is a sign of maturity and self-awareness!

What will your *analysis* be and how is this presented? Any *objectives* need to be relevant and achievable. We tend to use the criteria in the DFG legislation, even if the funding doesn't come via this funding stream. This supports the aim of equity of tenure – so home ownership doesn't impact on access to adaptations. (While something to aim for, it is unlikely that you can achieve true equity, as **homeowners** are expected to fund shortfalls in funding, and landlords can decline recommended adaptations.) **Objectives** could be:

- Access to and within the dwelling.

- Access to a family room.

- Access to a room to sleep in.

- Access to a toilet, bath, shower, etc., or provision of a room for these.

- Facilitating the preparation of food by the disabled person.

- Improving or providing a suitable heating system to meet the disabled person's needs, or facilitating the use of a source of power (gas/electric/oil/solar).

- Adaptations enabling the disabled person to care for someone dependent on them.

- Making the dwelling safe for the disabled person and others in the household.

- Facilitating access to and from a garden, or making a garden safe.

There are differences between the four nations of the UK so you will need to ensure you are applying the correct legislation and criteria in writing up your objectives (see Chapter 6).

Writing your identified needs and intended outcomes

The level of detail needed is team- and area-specific, so here we provide a general framework supporting the articulation of analysis and objectives:

- *Identified need:* It is easy to say that someone needs a ramp, but please allow us to challenge this approach. This is actually the *action* and not the *need*. Yes, they may need a ramp to exit the property, but think of the bigger picture – what will the provision of a ramp achieve? Will it support independence or enable a caregiver to safely assist someone out of their home? The need is actually the ability to enter and exit the dwelling and to access the community.

- *Proposed action:* This is the method of meeting the identified need. Keeping with the theme of access, this could be recommending ramped access to the front door.

- *Professional reasoning:* This is your evidence for the action you are proposing. Provision of a ramp may enable independent access for a wheelchair user, or a permanent ramp may be needed to enable use of a powered wheelchair. Alternatively, the ramp may support a caregiver to manoeuvre the wheelchair with reduced risk of injury.

In this section include evidence of observed environmental barriers such as steps or thresholds, as well as a person's occupational barriers.

- *Intended outcome of your recommendation:* We return to the 'bigger picture' for this one. Try to consider more than the immediate result of this change. Yes, they can enter and leave their home more safely, but what does this give them in terms of their life? Appropriate access in and out of a home can promote socialization, and enable access to education, work, health and leisure.

As occupational therapy is an **evidence-based profession**, this needs to be included in your reports and case notes. Evidence can be from the person's lived experience, information they (or you) have gathered from written resources and your previous experience. If you are aware of any practice guidelines, policies and research to support your reasoning, then use this. It may not go in your assessment or recommendation, but include it in your case notes and bring it up in supervision!

The report has now been written and shared with those who need to see it. Different services will vary, some adopting an approach where the person receives a copy of all correspondence, and others where it is held on file.

Next actions

Actions need to be agreed with the person you are supporting. These (and other options) may have been discussed at the assessment visit, but more as an outline of what may be considered. With experience, it becomes easier to identify next actions. There may be factors that prevent a proposed action being achieved, and you must not make promises you can't keep. If you have assured the person that it will happen, expectations have been raised. Therein lies a pathway to a complaint!

The next steps will depend on a number of factors. If you are *unsure of your next actions*, help is available. Your first line of support is from team members, either your peers or supervisor. It could be that you ask someone to read over your assessment report and then review options you have both identified. Alternatively, you could describe the situation and discuss your reasoning. Some teams have case discussion sessions built into the working week; these can be useful as you have access to a wide range of experience. It isn't advisable to ask a whole series of colleagues, though, as you risk confusing yourself with a wide range of opinions. Discussion must be documented in case records, as this will form part of your process of professional reasoning.

Another source of support is the relevant officer from the *district council* or *housing authority*. For simplicity we use the title 'grants officer', but depending on the range of responsibilities they hold, and the team they are affiliated with, titles will vary. Discussing the situation with the grants officer may mean a general discussion about the type of property and the options this affords, or it could be a more technical discussion about how to achieve an identified outcome. An alternative is to complete a scoping visit to the property that will enable you to discuss barriers and options to resolve them prior to submitting a recommendation. This will assist in ensuring that recommendations reflect what is achievable, but isn't required in every case.

Alternative sources of support are available on the internet, including:

- *DLF factsheets* (general advice on a range of daily living equipment): https://livingmadeeasy.org.uk/dlf-factsheets.

- *Foundations* (the national body for DFGs and Home Improvement Agencies in England): www.foundations.uk.com.

Creating a **scale drawing** from your sketch drawing can assist with your thought processes, especially where you need to ensure that equipment such as a bed will fit, or where you need to factor in the size of a turning circle.

To create a scale drawing you will need:

- Your sketch drawing.

- Paper – plain or graph.

- Pencil (and eraser!).

- A metric scale ruler (triangular or flat).

- Patience, and a sense of humour.

First, select the **scale** for your drawing. This will depend on the size of the room to be drawn up, your paper and the detail you need. The choice between graph paper and plain is a personal one. Graph paper offers ease of calculation, with lines already marked and clear right angles, but some find this distracting and prefer to use plain paper.

Creating a scale drawing uses the same process as your sketch drawing (just with more accuracy):

- Identify the appropriate scale.

- Draw the outline of the room.

- Add in the key features.

- Label them.

- Note the relevant measurements.[2]

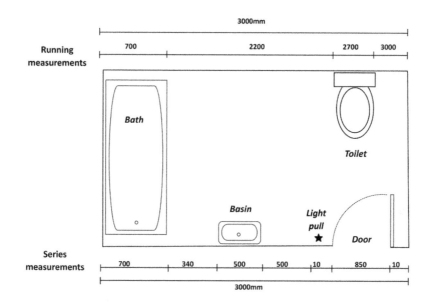

FIGURE 3. RUNNING AND SERIES MEASUREMENTS
Source: Ruth Parker

Rehousing

When it is not possible to adapt a property, rehousing must be considered. For most people this will be a highly charged decision, encompassing emotional and practical aspects.

Reasons for needing to relocate to another property include:

- Inability to achieve the required adaptation due to the property layout or construction.

- Costs exceeding the available budget.

- Landlord or property owner withholding consent.

---

2   You can either use running or series measurements (see Figure 3). Running measurements are totalled up as they are drawn in along each side of the plan. Series measurements have each individual measurement added in turn; when added together they total the full length of the wall. Series measurements provide more context for occupational therapy interventions.

- Choice by the person or the family to look for different accommodation.

- Social housing provider policy may be to rehouse tenants rather than adapt properties, considering this as more appropriate use of housing stock.

If a decision is made to seek rehousing, your role does not end there. If purchasing a property is under consideration, you can assist decision-making by completing an environmental assessment (subject to your team's remit and vendor agreement) (see the Appendix). The same support is appropriate for private rental properties. In both scenarios you will be able offer advice and information on suitability for adaptation and types of adaptation needed. This information will enable tenants and landlords to reach informed decisions, as landlords can consider the level of adaptation they can agree to.

For those moving into **social housing**, your role in assessing a property has the same purpose. It allows the provider to understand if the property offered is the best fit for the person or family, or if they need to consider other options in their housing portfolio. For this visit you may find that the housing officer will discuss potential adaptations in more detail, and may make a decision on the day as to the property's suitability.

Two notes of caution with supporting rehousing for those moving into social housing. First, timescales – there are usually key performance indicators that apply to empty or 'void' properties with an expectation that a new tenant is allocated the property in the shortest practical time. This may mean you need to complete an environmental assessment at short notice, and the potential tenant may feel under pressure to sign a lease. In this scenario it is usually accepted that any decision awaits the completion of your report. If your evaluation is that the property is not suitable, the tenant is not disadvantaged. We recommend that you ensure that your report is completed in a timely manner, however, so decisions can be made.

The second thing to consider is the role of the housing provider representative accompanying you on the visit. Do they have a role that enables them to make the necessary decisions? Some organizations separate the roles of housing allocation officer and adaptations officer. It is not unknown for a housing officer to assure a future tenant that the property can and will be adapted, only for the adaptations officer to decide that the scheme is impractical. As tenancy contracts often state, if signed, the tenant is confirming that they waive the right to request to move again.

It is always sensible to summarize the options discussed at the end of a visit and then follow this up with a brief email confirming if any adaptations have been agreed in principle. This gives an audit trail; should there be uncertainty in the future, you have evidence of any discussions.

Submitting recommendations

Teams will usually have a format for submitting a recommendation that helps with organizing the information you will provide, but what is the key information required?

- *The person:* Information provided needs to paint a picture rather than just a list of diagnoses. What you request for a child will differ to what is needed for an adult in their 70s. Usually, a description of their functional abilities is more appropriate than a diagnosis. Stating someone has a diagnosis of cerebral palsy does not provide a reflection of their functional ability; it is a descriptor for a group of conditions, and has the potential for misconception of the person's presentation. Giving the name of a rare genetic condition such as Adrenoleukodystrophy is ineffective. Consider the impact of the information you are sharing. A diagnosis is privileged information and only shared when essential. Would you want this level of information about your personal circumstances shared? A functional description is more useful: 'X is a full-time wheelchair user who is able to complete standing transfers unaided' illustrates more than a diagnosis.

- *The address to be adapted:* This is not as obvious as it seems. Most properties will be the current residence, but in some instances, such as for rehousing or property purchases, you will be seeking to adapt a property prior to someone living there or to reduce a delay once they move in. In these circumstances recommendations are usually only accepted once a tenancy agreement has been signed or contracts exchanged. Other information to include is the tenure or ownership of the property. This could be owner-occupied, social housing (council or housing association) or private rental. Confirming the property owner identifies the appropriate funding stream and who needs to be involved with providing necessary permissions. Briefly describe the property, including the number of bedrooms, previous adaptations and the type of construction, if known.

- *The household:* Knowing the household composition assists decision-making around use of rooms. This is also an opportunity to highlight if others in the household have their own additional needs.

- *Occupational issues/barriers experienced:* These are the issues you intend to resolve. Using the funding criteria provides the framework to articulate this, such as access to the property, safety, suitable heating system, and so on.

- *Adaptation(s) required:* These are the proposed solutions to the identified issues. The amount of detail required can differ between teams, services and authorities. You may only need to say 'ramped access to the front entrance', or more detail may be expected, such as the gradient, width of the ramp, size of platform, upstands and rails. Don't forget additional items such as **fused spurs** or changes to lights that facilitate provision of equipment. You may have access to standardized templates to provide necessary details. These are useful aide-mémoires as well as for providing information. A copy must be attached to the person's record to evidence your actions.

- *Intended outcomes:* Not all recommendation pro formas will ask for this, but providing this information can assist with evaluating the effectiveness of your recommendation and the completed adaptation. Did it achieve what you set out to do? Stating what you intend the adaptation to enable helps the person reading your request understand what you are asking for.

- *Solutions considered/tried:* It may be that you have tried or discounted several options, for example asking for a level-access shower. Demonstrating why a bath lift and over-bath shower haven't worked, or why these were discounted, supports an understanding of your recommendation.

- *Equipment provided/to be provided:* Adaptations are rarely the whole solution, and it is likely you will be providing equipment of some description. It may be that the equipment has already been provided and needs to be considered as part of the process. Alternatively, the adaptation enables equipment provision to address an identified need. Installation of items such as tracked hoists and a wall-mounted shower or changing bench needs appropriate construction for attachment points and fused spurs.

- *Additional information:* If there is something that you think is relevant, but which doesn't seem to fit in any of the boxes, make sure you include it – it all adds to the picture.

Some teams will have set pro formas to support recommendations for less complex adaptations such as grab rails and level-access showers. These are useful as aide-mémoires for the measurements you will need to take, as well as ensuring that your recommendation provides the level of detail needed. Figure 4 provides an example, with full-size examples available to download at https://library.jkp.com/redeem, using the code EDKQQWA.

Standard specification: grab rails
Bathroom

Installation of a plastic fluted grab rail to facilitate bathing.

Provide/provide and install (delete as required): **300mm / 450mm / 600mm** vertical grab rail.

Liaise with homeowner prior to install/advise prescriber if installation is not possible.

Vertical

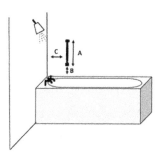

A: Length of grab rail (300mm / 450mm / 600mm)
B: Height from the edge of bath to centre of flange
C: Distance from wall to centre of grab rail

Service user's name	ID number	Address	Contact number
Other information			

Prescriber name	Date of request	Contact number	

FIGURE 4. STANDARD SPECIFICATION PRO FORMA
Source: Ruth Parker

Future planning

When you are making a recommendation, how far into the future should you plan for? For a child or young person, you should certainly be planning for adulthood, as you do not want to be revisiting every few years. Decisions and recommendations will be informed by your understanding of the person's diagnosis or disability. If you are aware a person has a degenerative condition with a clear prognosis, such as muscular dystrophy, then planning for full-time wheelchair use and hoist-assisted **transfers** is prudent. This may not mean the installation of a wash and dry toilet and ceiling track hoists straight away. Considering room layouts and locating load-bearing structures at the design stage, and fused spurs and power points in the specification, will reduce future disruption.

You may be supporting someone with a stable health condition, such as osteoarthritis, who may then experience a major change in their health, for example a traumatic amputation. You cannot plan for everything and may need to revise your assessment and recommendations. But you can extend your considerations beyond the barriers the person currently experiences. If they have difficulty managing the step to the front door but are negotiating stairs, suggesting a second stair rail is pragmatic.

Where you are working with a family, their vision of the size of their family may lead to difficult discussions. If they are planning a family of four and their second child has a disability, they may not want to utilize current 'spare' rooms to meet the need of this child. Unfortunately, you cannot work with intended outcomes that cannot be guaranteed. In a similar vein, you should not install toilet facilities to enable a toileting programme to be tried; you would need evidence that there is an awareness of needing the toilet before you can consider making a recommendation.

Conversely, you can unintentionally overprescribe – for example install-ing a stairlift for someone who is expected to require this level of support but who exceeds predictions. Provided the timescale isn't short between adaptation and independence, celebrate this positive outcome, and remem-ber that in the interim they will have needed the adaptation!

A note on electric sockets: if you think about how we live our lives today, the number of electric sockets provided in rooms, and bed-rooms especially, is never sufficient. Add to that someone who may spend a considerable amount of time in their bedroom – they will want to remain connected to the world, but may need to have a profiling bed, airflow mattress, feed pump, nebulizer and monitors. Add to these a light, phone charger, consoles and smart speaker. It is no surprise that people resort to extension leads, which are (a) not recommended and (b) trip hazards. A collaborative approach will enable you to understand how a person lives their life, and balance this with future equipment needs to predict appropriate provision... and maybe add an additional double socket!

Additional electric sockets may be requested simply to support provision of a profiling bed. This is a grey area, and you need to consider if the processes involved and the cost of the installation are worth it. If your role and remit is for specialist provision and you consider the RCOT's approach in *Adaptations without Delay* (2019), this can be considered 'universal provision', something someone can arrange themselves.

Of course, this isn't a blanket statement – a person's circumstances will direct your response. If they live in social housing, then the landlord should be approached; if they cannot afford the cost of an electrician or are in a vulnerable category, then you should be more proactive. A grant may not be the answer, but you do need to do your best to ensure that the works are carried out safely and by a qualified electrician.

Consider the equipment that goes into a room, both now and in the future. This is where your ability to create a scale drawing will come into its own, as it will allow you to try out different layouts and to check space for transfers and wheelchair mobility. It's not just the equipment at floor level to consider, however, as the pick-up and charge points for ceiling track hoists will also need to be identified. You really don't want to be lying in bed with the hoist charging above your head!

If the adaptation is for a child, consider their growth and development; equipment will get larger, but adults change shape too. If their stature places them close to exceeding the maximum dimensions of an item of equipment, consider that larger equipment may be needed. The equipment's safe working load and person's weight aids decision-making, and will highlight if additional structural strengthening is required.

In some areas applications to panels are required before adaptations are agreed, or panels are established to review complex adaptations. Members will vary dependent on the panel's terms of reference. The panel may consist of the grants officer, housing officer, occupational therapy representatives (adult and child teams) and technical officers. Some may require a case presentation, or a document review.

Your assessment is complete, and the recommendation has been submitted, so what's next?

Ideally a joint visit with the relevant grants or housing officer should be conducted. This will initiate a discussion with the person being supported, leading to an understanding of the current environment and what is required. From this, an initial proposal will be agreed. This could be specific, or, where a solution is not obvious, a more general proposal agreed. This, as options are considered and architectural plans created, develops into an appropriate solution.

Working with architectural plans

Architectural plans are key to successful communication during the adaptation process. Clutton *et al.* (2006) advise that they provide options, support decision-making and discussion, aid collaboration, reduce misunderstanding, manage expectations, define specific information and support successful outcomes. Although they can appear complex and confusing, the information they contain should set you on your way to becoming confident in using them.

Architectural plans are drawn up to support the identification and confirmation of the most appropriate solution. What do architectural plans look like? They vary: they can be hand drawn on paper, digital 2D drawings or 3D renders of a design. Who is the scheme designer? Considering the information in Chapter 4, a surveyor or architectural technician usually draws them up. A relatively recent development is the use of a contractor or designer. This is where the contractor decides on the most appropriate scheme and presents this, often for schemes such as installation of a level-access shower.

What are architectural plans for and what do they give us?

Architectural plans provide an accurate *visual representation of the discussions* held and the space this relates to. This is achieved through the use of a *scale* to ensure that all elements within the drawing are in proportion to each other in size and spatial orientation. This will be completed for the relevant portion of the property and drawn to scale. (It's unlikely that the full property will be drawn up unless the scheme is extensive.)

Architectural plans provide the necessary information for a particular scheme. If the changes are internal, such as to a bathroom layout, there is no need for a full ground floor layout, exterior representation or its location within its plot. These additional views are provided if the adaptation alters the exterior appearance, or, in the case of ramps and hardstanding, the land surrounding the property.

There are three common types of architectural drawings:

- *Site plans:* In the context occupational therapists are working in, site plans will usually be of the property and the land immediately surrounding it. Some may provide a wider view of the surrounding area, but this is more commonly part of a new-build scheme.

- *Plan:* This is the type of drawing occupational therapists usually work with, as seen in Figure 5. The drawing is in the horizontal plane, with this example providing the complete layout of the home (and it is used for case studies in Chapter 24 later).

- *Elevation:* Elevations show the face of the building – the vertical plane (see Figure 6). This is what you will see if you are standing looking at the property. Often these are useful for people to visualize the change to their home. We are used to looking at our homes this way, and not everyone can make sense of the information provided in a plan view, especially when there are significant alterations to the internal layout.

Architectural drawings will represent the current situation (existing layout) and then illustrate a solution (proposed layout), enabling you to evaluate the changes. (Note: Figures 5 and 6 only show the existing situation.)

There is a wealth of information contained within architectural drawings, and we start with the title block (see Figure 7). All sets of drawings will include a title block, and while it may not appear to have any relevance to proposed adaptations, you do need to pay attention to the detail it provides.

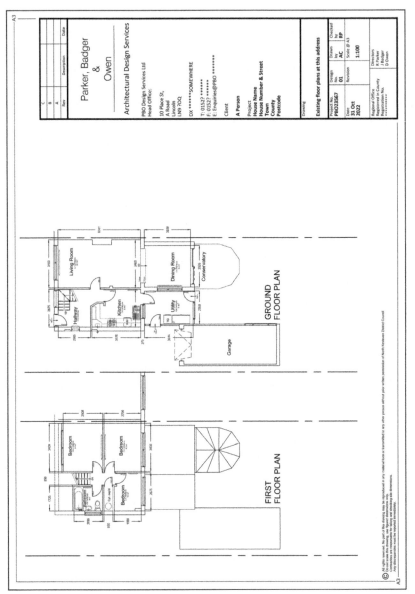

FIGURE 5. ARCHITECTURAL DRAWING, PLAN VIEW
Source: North Kesteven District Council/Andrea Cox

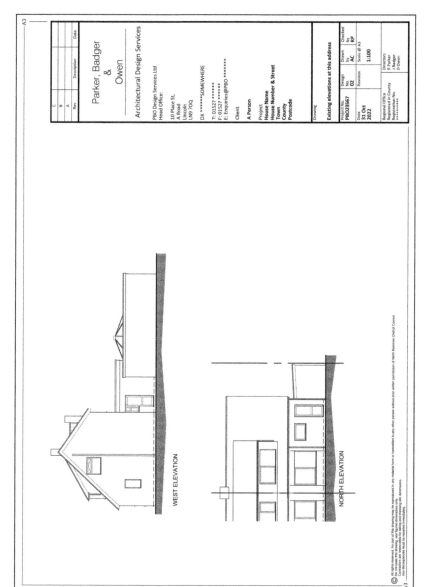

FIGURE 6. ARCHITECTURAL DRAWING, ELEVATION VIEW
Source: North Kesteven District Council/Andrea Cox

Rev	Description	Date
C		
B		
A		

Parker, Badger & Owen

Architectural Design Services

PBO Design Services Ltd
Head Office:

10 Place St,
A Road
Lincoln
LN9 ?OQ

DX ******SOMEWHERE

T: 0152? ******
F: 0152? ******
E: Enquiries@PBO *******

Client

A Person

Project
House Name
House Number & Street
Town
County
Postcode

Drawing

Existing floor plans at this address

Project No. **PBO23567**	Design No. **01**	Drawn by **AC**	Checked by **RP**
Date **31 Oct 2022**	Revision	Scale @ A3 **1:100**	

Regional Office Registered in County Registration No. **********	Directors R Parker J Badger D Owen

FIGURE 7. TITLE BLOCK
Source: North Kesteven District Council/Andrea Cox

Within the title block we see the detail of the company or organization responsible for producing the architectural drawing. The title block includes:

1. Contact details – essential for communication, discussion and clarification of queries!

2. The address.

3. The person the plans have been drawn for – the service user/client/patient, depending on your service's terminology.

4. The location to be adapted.

5. What this drawing is of (essential when there are several rooms or areas illustrated).

6. The reference number for the project – this will be consistent across all sets of drawings.

7. The design number.

8. The initials of the person responsible for the drawing.

9. If applicable, the initials of the person who has checked or reviewed the drawing.

10. The date the drawing is created – this will assist with checking if this drawing is the most recent iteration.

11. The scale of the drawing, and the paper size required to print it to the correct scale.

12. The revision to the scheme that this drawing relates to referenced by a letter and a date.

Why is all this important? As the detail of the drawing changes, you will need to know what these changes are so you can track them and understand how these impact on other areas. When an agreement on a scheme is reached, you need to know which version of the architectural drawings this is based on.

This may seem like common sense, but life is never simple when you are working across disciplines and organizations. Although the intention is always to maintain communication, sometimes things slip. Someone may ask to include 'a small change' that the person creating the drawings sees as a simple addition with little impact. This is not always the case, and it is often the occupational therapist who must then think creatively.

Would the changes listed below make a significant difference to a scheme? Consider these scenarios and then see if your thoughts align with the outcomes.

(a) Altering the swing of a door from into the family room to into the bedroom.

(b) Adding a loft access hatch.

(c) Altering a set of French doors from the left-hand side, opening first to the right.

(d) Installation of a 'standard'-height toilet.

(a) It was agreed the tracked hoist charge point would be located to the side of the doorway. Altering the direction of swing resulted in the door colliding with the spreader bar on opening, damaging the paintwork and preventing the door from being opened quietly. The parents raised this as an issue, requesting charge point relocation. Reviewing the record revealed the parents requested the change after scheme finalization. The parents had discussed alterations with the grants officer and contractor, but it was considered 'so minor' that they did not believe it necessary to involve the occupational therapist. Suffice to say the request to reconfigure the tracked hoist layout was declined, and it was recommended that the parents employ a joiner to alter the door to the agreed specification.

(b) Adding a loft hatch to provide access to the void above a new extension seems a practical response. Not so if the location is directly in line with the hoist track, as agreed on a site visit with the contractor, surveyor and the tracked hoist installer. The drawings for the hoist had been shared. The hoist was installed in a slightly different location, but this caused issues with transfer points for both the bed and the bath. After a number of years the scheme was revisited, the bath resited and the track layout revised – frustrating and costly!

(c) French doors will have a leaf selected for installation of the lock, and this is used as the main entry and exit point. The second leaf generally remains fixed and is only opened as required. Alteration to the locking side was made as the homeowner and contractor agreed 'doors of this type should always have the right-hand side as the lock side', differing from the specification. The adaptation was created within restricted space for someone with complex health needs. French doors were provided facilitating ramped access via the left-hand leaf. The issue was that there was insufficient space at the end of the bed for wheelchair access. The person could not reach the opening leaf, unnecessarily increasing dependence on others in order to leave the property. It was essential to alter the door configuration.

(d) As occupational therapists prescribe adaptations to meet the needs of an individual, recommendations are tailored to meet assessed needs. This can be identifying a specific height, length or width. In this case, a lower toilet height was specified for someone with restricted growth. The change to a 'standard'-height toilet was made by a contractor without consultation, and only identified at scheme completion. A usable space was delayed as the specified toilet had to be ordered and installed.

How do these relate to the title block, as none of the information specifying these key details is included in the block itself? Unpicking the situation, in each case it was the date and revision information that enabled identification of what had been agreed and where changes had been made but not confirmed. For (c), the contractor and homeowner consulted a set of drawings that pre-dated the agreed scheme and did not include revisions to the door set.

Since the COVID-19 pandemic, working patterns have changed, and there is a far higher reliance on video and telephone calls rather than site visits. It's always best to check before starting an in-depth discussion that the architectural drawings discussed are the ones that you have had sight of, and the easiest way of doing this is to check both the date of the drawing and the revision reference.

Moving on, consider *scale* and *paper size*. We no longer expect physical copies of architectural drawings – better for the planet and in line with electronic case management. This does, however, require you to take note of both scale and paper size provided in the title block. The benefits of digital copies include wider access and the ability to review and discuss these when working remotely.

If you are sent paper copies, our advice is to scan and save them, but note that these will not be to scale in this format. Figures 5 and 6 show that the drawings are to scale when printed at A3.

KEY SKILLS FOR HOUSING ADAPTATIONS

Architectural drawings may be presented using different scales, such as 1:100 for elevation drawings, as in the examples provided. Where more detail is required, it is common for 1:50 or 1:20 to be used, but always check. Looking at a scale ruler you can see a whole range of scales to choose from. Remember that measurements will be given in millimetres.

When printing drawings, check that the printer settings will result in an accurate copy. Some printers have a print 'as original' setting but default to a 'best fit' setting. This will give you an image that is slightly smaller than the scale stated.

If you are sent drawings that are scaled to 1:50 on A1 paper but you can only print to A3, with patience, a photocopier and a scale ruler, you can resolve this. The image size can be altered via the zoom function – you will need to play around a bit to get the result you need, but it is worth it. Zoom in and then compare a given dimension with a scale ruler; once you have an image that corresponds to the correct scale, you are good to go. To save the effort of repeating this process at a later date, make additional copies and note the corresponding scale.

So far we have looked at plans and elevation, title block and working with different scales, but we have not yet discussed how to interpret drawings. Architectural drawings can include detail of the fabric of the building, utilities and a level of detail beyond the scope of your recommendation. We will try and guide you to the key details you will be using.

Architectural symbols

Architectural symbols are icons used to indicate features and details within a drawing, and remove the need to use labels that clutter up drawings, making interpretation difficult. Many symbols used are easy to interpret, but others may not be quite so obvious (see Figure 8). Have a look at these and see how many you recognize.

Knowledge check: what do these symbols represent? ★

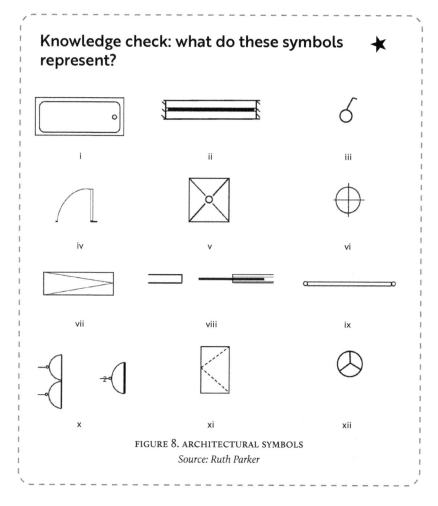

FIGURE 8. ARCHITECTURAL SYMBOLS
Source: Ruth Parker

There are differences between the UK and other countries, but also with icons used by different professionals. There are resources on the internet with lists of different icons. If you are really stuck, however, just ask – it's better to be certain than operate on assumptions.

How do you think you got on with the icons shown in Figure 8? It's easier when they are in context:

i) *A bath*, but not just any bath. This is rectangular and shows which end the waste (drain) is situated. This tells you it is not a corner or roll-top bath. Its position within a drawing will indicate if it is set into the corner of a room or if it fills available wall space.

ii) *Casement window*; this is the plan view and shows the width and location along the length of the wall. From this you cannot see the height of the window or the height at which it is inset in the wall.

iii) *A single-gang light switch*. The light fitting this relates to can only be operated from one position in the room. If there is a second short section (making it look more like a key), this is a two-gang light switch and can be operated from a second location. It is useful to know if the person enters their bedroom with the light on, and then switches it off once they are in bed. The drawing would need to show a two-gang light switch by both the door and bed.

iv) *An internal door*. From this you can see which room the door opens into and which side is hinged. When thinking about access consider doors as barriers when closed and open. If the direction of travel is towards the door leaf when it is opened, it adds another obstacle, so consider the impact of changing the hinge position. A note of caution: if this is on an existing door, consider the position of any light switches as you don't want to remove one barrier only to find the person can enter a room but can't switch on the light!

v) *A shower tray*. This one is square with a central waste (drain). The size and location of the tray (sometimes called a former) and waste will vary depending on the design. These enable you to identify if they meet need, and are compatible with equipment and shower head position. This is key when thinking about level-access showers as the direction of the water may mean that some will fall outside of the tray and may not flow towards the waste.

vi) *A pendant light fitting*. Traditionally in the UK these are installed centrally (or closer to a window in the case of bedrooms). If you want to install a tracked hoist – especially an H frame system, you need to consider if this is the most appropriate position or lighting type.

vii) *A ramp*. The triangle indicates an upward slope from the wide base of the triangle to its apex. There should be a platform or level area at the base and top of the ramp. (An alternative indicator is an arrow showing gradient direction, but check that there is an annotation identifying if this is up or down.)

viii) *A pocket door*. This is a sliding door set within a stud wall rather than along the face of a wall. This icon represents a single leaf pocket door, but there are systems allowing for two door leaves to slide back at the same time. This enables the creation of a suitable opening where space on side walls is limited. The advantage of pocket doors is that wall space remains. Wall-hung sliding doors need their direction of travel kept clear.

ix) *Radiator*. This icon indicates width and room position only. Height, depth, thermostatic valve position and thermal output are not indicated.

x) *Two symbols that mean the same thing: an internal double power outlet* (electric socket). This symbol works logically: if there is only one dome, it is a single socket etc. Regulations specify height installation, so you can presume for newer properties or when planning an extension that this will be at approximately 1000mm from floor level. For any other building you will not be able to tell how high these are from the plans. As your designs are tailored for individuals you can ask for flexibility. If someone mobilizes by 'commando crawling' and prefers to be floor-based for activities and occupations, then requesting electric sockets at a lower level responds to assessed need.

xi) *Casement window* (hinged on left-hand side). This symbol appears similar to the ramp symbol but would be seen in an *elevation* drawing. The apex of the triangle indicates the hinge position – usually left-, right- or top-hung windows. Tilt- and turn-type windows have a second triangle overlaid to indicate the two options for opening.

xii) *A recessed spotlight*. This icon is similar to the pendant light but with the crossed lines on the diagonal. This should not be confused with a recessed downlight.

Let's revisit the drawings in Figures 5 and 6 (you can view and download larger copies online at https://library.jkp.com/redeem, using the code EDKQQWA).

Knowledge check

1. Can you identify which of the windows on the plan view is the top opening window shown in the elevation? Which room is this window in?

2. Which rooms are separated by a change in level? Which is higher?

3. How many external doors are there?

4. How many radiators are there?

5. What divides the dining room and the conservatory?

(Answers are provided at the end of the chapter.)

So far, we have looked at plans and elevation, scale and paper size and architectural icons. These will all help you interpret drawings in relation to the needs of the person you are supporting.

What is it you should be looking for?

Access points and routes:

- How is the property and outside space accessed?

- What are the routes between essential rooms?

- How are additional floors accessed?

Use of rooms:

- Can you identify which occupations are completed in which rooms or areas?

- Which rooms should you focus on?

Personal care:

- What spaces are available for personal care tasks?

- What options are there in place for bathing or showering?

- Where are toilets located?

Household tasks:

- Who prepares the meals and who is responsible for laundry?

- Who maintains the outside space?

Leisure and socialization:

- Are there defined spaces for shared meals and family time?

- Does the outdoor space enable activities?

- Can the person access activities outside of the home if they wish to do so?

Once you understand the layout and space represented in the architectural drawing, it is time to apply your knowledge and understanding of the person's situation:

- What are the barriers and enablers you identify? It can be easy to focus on the negative, so begin with a strengths-based approach – not only for the person, but also their home.

- What aspects of the home support the person's meaningful occupations, activities and relationships? Be aware of these, so when addressing identified needs and barriers you don't inadvertently remove these enablers.

Consideration of assessed needs identifies the aspects of the home that present barriers. This is where you compare the existing property and proposed layout. Working through each of the needs and barriers you can evaluate the proposed changes and the impact they are likely to have – both as enablers and as potential barriers.

Some key features to consider are:

- Functionality and usability of ramps – space at entry and exit points.

- Door widths and direction of swing.

- Position of doors and windows – impact on placement of furniture.

- Location and size of turning circles in essential rooms.

- 'Pinch points' that could limit movement.

- Transfer space – are these the correct side of a bed for the method used?

- Lighting and heating – location, control and type.

- Bath – type and location of taps.

- Shower – type, location of control and shower head.

- Power and charging points – location and number.

This is not an exhaustive list as every situation is unique. The role of the occupational therapist is to take available information, apply it to the proposal, and through a process of review, discussion and revision, identify the most suitable solution.

You have now received your first set of drawings and reviewed them. Have all needs been met? Have you discussed and agreed the drawings with the person you are supporting? Perfect – you can respond advising that you are satisfied with the proposed scheme. If you review the drawings and issues remain or new barriers are created, you will need to advise the person responsible for the drawings that additional revisions are required.

This review and revision process continues until a suitable scheme is achieved. How much you involve the person whose property is being adapted will vary. (Think of the 'ladder of participation'…) If a scheme is proposed and you can see that there are several major revisions, it may not be appropriate to share this with anyone. It may be better to wait until you have a more realistic scheme – but do keep the person updated, as there is nothing worse than a long silence while waiting for information.

This scenario presumes that the drawings are commissioned by the local authority or housing provider. If the person has opted to commission their own drawings, it is expected that they will receive copies of all versions.

It is not possible to predict how long this review and revision process will take as it is affected by the work capacity of all involved, the number of revisions and length of discussions.

Once all parties agree the scheme, the next step varies, dependent on a range of factors:

- Is the work to be completed in-house? This removes the need for a tender process.

- Does the scheme have to go out to tender? This means that several building contractors have the opportunity to submit quotes to complete the scheme. Standard schedules of work may apply, reducing the need to negotiate costs. Contractors may choose to submit a quote based only on the schedule of works. Where a set schedule does not apply, the contractor will need to complete a site visit to understand the scope of the work to prepare a quote.

- Is planning permission required? If works are small in scale and internal to the property, it is less likely planning permission is needed. External works may fall within permitted development[3] and can proceed without a planning application. If a planning application is required, expect that this process will take at least 12 weeks. The progress of applications can be tracked via the planning authority's portal.

As we write, the pandemic is fresh in our memory, along with Brexit and the war in Ukraine – all impacting manufacturing and supply chains. In response to this, many areas are requiring contractors to guarantee that all necessary building materials are available prior to starting work. This may add a further delay to the process, but it is a prudent approach.

---

3   There are exceptions to the requirement to request planning permission. Dependent on the size and height of an extension, it may fall within this category. Different exceptions are applied, such as if there has already been an increase in the footprint of a property, or if it falls within a conservation area.

Once the scheme has been agreed and a contractor has been appointed, who (hopefully) has given a start date in the not-too-distant future, it's time for the pre-start meeting.

Pre-start meeting

Often a pre-start meeting is held to discuss the practical aspects of the scheme. Attendees usually include the person whose property is to be adapted, the grants, technical or housing officer, contractor and occupational therapist. This is an opportunity to confirm the length of time that the build will take, key timescales, and when it is appropriate for the occupational therapist to arrange surveys for equipment (aiming for provision to coincide with the build completion). This is an ideal time for key aspects to be confirmed, such as where walls and ceilings need strengthening, the direction of fall from the shower head and service connections.

This meeting will enable the person to ask questions about the build process. These could be quite technical as they seek to understand the changes to be made to their home. If there are to be disruptions to essential services, when these will be and how long they last for will be key lines of enquiry, especially in cases where there is a direct risk to a person's health and wellbeing such as a nebulizer, feed pump or airflow mattress. Often there is a level of anxiety about the process, so questions could focus on basic details such as, what time will the contractor be on site? Where will they park? How will access to toilet facilities be maintained?

If an adaptation is being completed for someone with high levels of anxiety, a learning disability or neurodivergence, it may be that those working on site will have to be mindful of their approach and interactions. For those with behaviours that challenge, the need to prevent access to tools and building materials may be required, or additional vigilance over exit points from the house and garden.

You will be preparing for the point at which the adaptation will be used, which means assessing for any equipment that will be needed. This may mean ordering a shower chair to arrive ready for completion, or a survey for installation of a tracked hoist or height-adjustable shower or changing bench. This means that you need to coordinate surveys, quotes and orders and allow for lead times (the time between placing an order and the delivery or installation date). Communication and coordination with contractors is essential to achieve this!

Scheme completion

Your role continues once the adaptation is complete. Depending on the processes in place it may be that a post-completion visit is required to 'sign off' the adaptation. The concept of Post-Occupancy Evaluation means obtaining feedback on completion of construction projects including use of the building and user satisfaction – a more formal process than post-completion visits, but effectively one with the same aim.

This is an opportunity for you to discuss how the person for whom the adaptation was completed feels about what has been achieved and the process by which it was achieved. At this point it is important to take the time to listen and understand their position if they feel that the end result or the process was less than satisfactory.

A snagging visit should have been completed by the relevant officer, who will liaise with the contractor to agree how any issues raised will be addressed. If they haven't been addressed by the time of your post-completion visit, we recommend you reference these in your case notes. It may not be your responsibility to ensure they are resolved, but if you have an ongoing involvement with the person, you can support them in ensuring they are followed up.

In your evaluation of the completed adaptation consider if the intended outcomes have been achieved. To do this, revisit your initial recommendation to confirm stated objectives. Discussion with the person you are supporting and your observations will enable you to (hopefully) confirm that the outcomes are positive. But what if the adaptation hasn't achieved what you intended? What are your next steps? Do not presume that the whole thing has been a disaster and that you got it wrong!

First, discuss how the adaptation is used – it may be that the person hasn't adjusted to a new way of using the space. We tend to stick to familiar routines, but the changes made may need a new approach to activities. Revisit the recommendation: did you state a level threshold? Is that what was provided? Sometimes there are misunderstandings or miscommunications. Methodically working through what was requested, the scheme of works and the completed adaptation can highlight where issues originated. As mentioned before, changes can be made during the course of a build. These may be in response to issues identified as building work progresses or because they were thought to be a 'good idea'.

A **DFG recommendation** was made to create an additional bedroom to enable two teenage boys to have their own space, responding to their complex medical needs and to support their parents in providing care. The scheme was expanded to include a bedroom and an en suite for their paternal grandmother, who was no longer able to live independently and who self-funded this work. This meant that there would be five bedrooms in the property.

The occupational therapist visited following completion of the adaptation, and realized that there were only four bedrooms. When this was raised with the family, they advised that the contractor had suggested incorporating the smallest bedroom into the bathroom to provide a more generous space and a larger bed/sitting room for the grandmother. This meant that the two boys had to continue to share a bedroom, and the family advised that they were happy with this arrangement. What would you do in this scenario? Is this okay? What would your next steps be?

The issue is, the recommendation specified both teenagers would have their *own* bedrooms, and this had not been achieved. Although the family had part-funded the works and were satisfied with the outcome, the occupational therapist had to advise the recommendation for adaptation had not been met. Following discussions and review of the works it was decided that they did not meet the terms of the DFG. Either the family had to self-fund the scheme, or the contractor had to revise the scheme in line with the schedule of works.

It may be that when you visit, the snagging list has not been resolved. Ideally there will be no areas that need revision, but realistically there often are. Any negative response to the change may simply reflect a person's wish to regain their home and their control over it.

If the adaptation process has taken a significant length of time, the person's needs may have changed, either because they have a degenerative condition or their health may have deteriorated due to a new condition. This will require a reassessment.

If there is an extended period between stages of the adaptation, the person may contact you for updates. Would it be more appropriate for them to contact the grants or housing officer directly? Occupational therapists should, wherever possible, be empowering people. At times the emphasis on maintaining lines of communication may not work in your favour and actually increase your workload.

A final note to this chapter: Occupational therapists are often the hub for communication throughout the adaptation process, but this does not mean that they are the only people to provide information and updates. Revisiting previous advice, occupational therapists shouldn't be providing an update if a recommendation for adaptation is declined. The decision lies with the district council, local authority or housing provider, who are best placed to provide the reasoning for their decision.

This chapter has been lengthy, with much to assimilate, demonstrating that your role in the adaptation is complex and multi-faceted. Understanding these key skills will provide a firm foundation from which to expand your expertise, develop competence and build confidence.

Answers to the knowledge check

1. Which room is this window in? *Bathroom.*

2. Which rooms are separated by a change in level? Which is higher? *Living and dining room; dining room is higher.*

3. How many external doors are there? *Three.*

4. How many radiators are there? *Three.*

5. What divides the dining room and the conservatory? *Sliding door.*

8

Design for a Diverse Population: Cultural Considerations in Practice

Knowledge check

Reflect on the following questions:

* Do you consider your knowledge and experience is wide enough to appreciate the impact of culture and belief in the lives of those you are supporting?

* Does your culture or belief system influence the adaptations you recommend?

* Are there any areas in which you feel you need to expand your knowledge?

How you approach those you interact with sets the tone for your future working relationship, and ultimately affects how identified needs are met. You are entering a person's private and intimate space, somewhere that reflects their view of the world. You are (in the context of this book) looking to make changes to this environment, and therefore understanding what is important to them will inform future conversations.

Although this chapter focuses on culture and belief, it is important to also consider ableism. Your role and remit is to minimize the impact of disability, and you need to be aware of your own attitude and approach, both to those you support and also those you work with.[1] Be aware of and call out bias (including your own), avoid only focusing on visible disabilities, and cease using terms such as 'struggling' or 'bravery'.[2] For RCOT members, the September 2022 *OT News* article 'Let's change how we talk about disability' (McDonald 2022) places this in the context of occupational therapy.

It is important to consider the cultures and beliefs of those you are working with. The UK's multi-cultural and multi-faith society means that in professional practice you will be working with people and families whose way of life may differ from your own. These differences may not be linked to race or religion, but could simply be something you are not familiar with or wouldn't give a second thought to.

> A note to consider: Not all who list a faith or ethnicity will be devout or will have adopted or retained cultural traits. Do not make presumptions either way.

Sometimes something as simple as checking if someone would prefer you to remove your shoes before you enter their property can make a significant difference. You may have grown up in a household where outdoor footwear is worn indoors without comment, but for some, this will cause distress or discomfort. Be sensitive and understand where you may cause offence, but also how you can build good working relationships right from the first contact you have with people.

This chapter is not designed to inform you about all the different aspects of a culture or a belief system you may need to consider. This is impossible, and, to be honest, destined to fail. Henley and Schott (1999, p.378) highlight that writing in this area is 'a fine balance between what may be useful information and damaging generalisations'. The intention is to highlight some aspects, encourage you to increase your awareness, and to make this an integral part of your practice.

We have gathered together information, from our experiences and from online sources, educating ourselves in the process but in no way presenting this as the definitive guide. To this end the information in this chapter is not

---

1   Occupational therapy voices in this area include @GeorgiaVineOT (author of *Occupational Therapy, Disability Activism, and Me: Challenging Ableism in Healthcare*, scheduled for publication April 2024, Jessica Kingsley Publishers), @AbleOTUK and @DisruptOT.
2   A useful blog providing some additional information and context is available at: https://affinot.co.uk/2022/09/22/language-and-discrimination-by-natalie-hicks-nataliehixy

divided into sections according to a culture or belief system, but grouped around activities and actions – ours, and those we are working with.

The first tool you have is yourself. Reading this chapter is a start, but you can identify some of the information you need in the referral and initial assessment. Educating yourself about the key days and dates in the relevant calendar will help with planning visits (online calendars with key celebrations are available). Be reflective, understanding your own beliefs and attitudes. Do these colour your approach and recommendations? Are you imposing your 'norm' on others?

You may not consider superstitions to have any relevance to your life, but for others they may guide their approach, from not agreeing to a visit on Friday the 13th or having issues if works require a ladder over an access point. Not all belief systems are linked to a faith – an example of this is Feng Shui, which may have implications on how adaptations are designed.

Do not be dismissive, and take time to discuss and listen to others, although there may need to be a compromise on both sides to ensure the planned outcome can be achieved.

Planning visits

The process of an adaptation will begin with a visit, an initial assessment or a rehousing or environmental assessment. Planning this, taking into consideration significant calendar dates, will assist in the instigation of a good working relationship. Initial information-gathering to understand how a family lives includes sensitive topics reflecting cultural norms.

Food and nutrition

Food and nutrition are key to good health, but they are also opportunities to socialize, and have cultural or religious links. The kitchen is often described as the 'heart of the home'. For some, their role and identity are intrinsically linked to this area of the home and family life. While many are happy to adapt to having ready meals, these do not necessarily meet cultural needs associated with shared meals. There are clear links between religious beliefs and food groups or meals, which includes fasting. Those who are fasting, for example, may prefer to avoid demonstration of issues that link to food preparation, such as a hot drink assessment.

Ensuring that the kitchen environment enables a person's role or mean-ingful occupation to continue will require different adaptations dependent on your assessment of need. Planning an adaptation may require understanding of how different food groups are stored and prepared, for example separation of milk and meat, and also cooking methods such as the use of a Tandoor.

A note to consider: For some cultures, the offering of food and drink to visitors is essential. This may challenge you, your beliefs or dietary needs, or impact the time available for a visit to be completed.

Personal care

The most frequent adaptations completed are ensuring access to bathing and personal care. In the UK our expectations around bathing have altered in the last 50 years, changing from a presumption that a bath was appropriate and not a daily requirement. Now showers and en-suite facilities are commonplace, and wet rooms are no longer viewed as a 'specialist' provision.

There is an expectation that bathing and personal hygiene should be completed in privacy and dignity. What this means to a person will vary; some people have grown up in a family where nudity and bodily functions are not considered a private topic, whereas others would find this level of openness distressing. This is one of those occasions where your own thoughts on the subject need to be placed to one side, supporting as far as possible the preference of the person you are supporting. There are compromises to be made – if someone cannot access bathing without support, but is unused to others seeing them naked, a way of meeting their needs appropriately will need to be identified.

Some practices are linked to practicality. Those raised in a hot climate or whose family practice stems from this type of culture may expect or wish to bathe more frequently. It may be that antiseptic is always added to bathwater, talc is used after bathing, or that there are separate towels and soap for the upper and lower body. Understanding this level of detail will assist in identifying which, if any, changes need to be made in the bathroom.

The discussion over bathing or showering is not just around practicality. Some belief systems require washing in running water before prayers are said, there are also cultural norms to be considered where a bath may be used, but with running water rather than filling the bath. This could be via a shower hose attachment or the use of a jug and bowl.

Other personal care activities need to be considered such as shaving, hair care and dental care, where teeth must be cleaned before and after every meal. Again, these activities are ones we all need to complete, but our routines will vary, as will the importance we place on their completion and the impact felt if they cannot be achieved.

Where bathing facilities are located differs – we don't all live in 'standard' accommodation. It was once commonplace to have a privy in the garden and to wash in front of the fire. But that's not to say everyone has the same bathroom access as you. En-suite facilities to the master bedroom are featured in many new homes and added to existing properties. Bathrooms aren't necessarily located on the same floor as the bedrooms, such as in some terraced properties or in external blocks, such as on Traveller or Gypsy sites.

Having conversations with people about their bathing habits and preferences sheds a light on activities that are rarely observed or discussed. These can be difficult for people to articulate or share. This increases when you start discussing toileting. Take a moment to consider how you feel about discussing bowel movements or menstruation outside of a medical consultation. The need to consider how personal intimate care activities are completed means you will have to initiate difficult conversations and complete these sensitively. It may be that this is not a conversation that can be had between members of the opposite sex, as for some cultures this is taboo.

How intimate personal cleanliness is maintained differs between cultures, belief systems and the way (and where) we are brought up. Take toilet design – we have a western concept of design, being a toilet that we sit on with waste flushed away. However, many cultures use a squat toilet, and both sit and squat designs can be wet (flush) or dry systems. Adapting to a different type of toilet may be a necessary adjustment that needs to be considered. You may also be requested to consider the orientation of a toilet in relation to the Qiblah.[3]

Moving on from the actual design, the method of cleaning after toilet use differs. For some the key aspect is the position of facilities promoting the use of a specific hand. Not all cultures use toilet paper to cleanse after toileting – water may be used from a jug or hose, or a bidet may be essential. Wash and dry toilets or bidet toilet seats are becoming mainstream provision and resolve many of the issues around personal intimate cleaning; however, traditional or observant Jews may not operate electrical devices on Shabbat (the Sabbath), for example, and so these may only be effective for part of the week.

---

3   Advice on this can be found at: https://islamqa.info/en/answers/69808/ruling-on-building-toilets-that-face-the-qiblah – this does advise that for indoor facilities this is not a concern, although the person you are supporting may have strong feelings on the subject. If they will not use a facility where they turn their back on the Qiblah, the direction towards the Kaaba in the Sacred Mosque in Mecca, it is pragmatic to design around this belief.

Where access to a toilet is not possible, a commode is the usual solution, but for many this is not an acceptable option. If there is resistance it may not just be that they dislike the idea, so again, further discussion and investigation is needed to identify a suitable solution.

Worship

Homes are locations for worship as well as for family life. Devotional activities may require access to running water prior to prayer, and there may be shrines located within the home. For some the kitchen has significance as the cleanest and purest room within the home, and may be the location for a shrine. It shouldn't need to be said, but treat these with respect. Moving a holy book for your convenience is not acceptable, and being aware of the position of items can be key, such as Lord Buddha being placed highest within a room.

There are dedicated spaces that need to be considered – you should ask permission prior to entering these, and you may be asked to remove your footwear. Spaces set aside for worship can be a conundrum, especially when occupational therapists' approach to adaptations is to consider the home as a whole. Identifying a space as suitable for adaptation where its use has such great significance is likely to be met with resistance.

Responsibility for decision-making

Being sensitive to how others live their lives includes how decisions are made. Who owns the property will affect decision-making, which means that the final decision is dependent on someone other than the person you are supporting. Also, unless someone lives alone, others will be affected by any changes you are recommending.

How decisions are reached can and will differ between families, but you do need to appreciate the processes by which they make decisions. In some cultures and families decisions are deferred to elders, to a patriarch or matriarch, or members of a specific gender. You may wish to have discussions with all relevant family members at the same time to hear all opinions. In some cultures this isn't possible, however, as there is separation between genders.

It may be expected that authority figures are deferred to. You may not recognize yourself in this way, but completing recommendations or proposing schemes may mean you are viewed as such. Therefore, be sure that an acceptance of what has been suggested is because the person and those they live with are actually in agreement that this is what is appropriate. Ensure their voice is both heard and listened to.

Working in this area it is reasonable that you will make decisions based on the evidence base you have access to and your experience. Be aware that while you can provide information to explain why a course of action is recommended, some people need thought and consideration through prayer before a decision can be made.

Personal space

Personal space is just that, something that is individual to each of us, but underpinned by the culture we grow up in. Posture, distance maintained, touch, as well as greetings differ between cultures. Consider the title used to address someone, and aspects such as if you should (or shouldn't) offer to shake hands on arrival or leaving, and proximity, for example sitting on the edge of a bed.

Although our awareness of other cultures is increased through television and film, seeing posture, eye contact and other non-verbal cues on screen is very different than during personal interactions. Some may view direct eye contact as inappropriate, but others may misinterpret not making eye contact as avoidance or deceit. Non-verbal cues or gestures differ across the globe – smiling may be used to indicate anger or discomfort rather than pleasure.

Communication

Working with people who may not be fluent in your native language (whatever that may be) may present difficulties in explaining what you are trying to achieve or to differentiate between different options. How you effectively communicate ideas may require support from others. Family members are often used, but this then introduces an imbalance as family dynamics come into play. Utilizing alternative methods to ensure comprehension and prevent bias may be needed. Online translation programmes can be useful, but do not presume literacy in any language.

It is worth noting that although you may hold conversations in English, meanings of words or phrases may differ. For example, in the UK the term *first floor* is used to identify the storey accessed by a flight of stairs from the ground floor, but in Canada and the USA, *first floor* refers to what in the UK is the *ground floor*. A miscommunication around this could have significant implications for the location of amenities.

Part of communication is how topics are presented for discussion. Within the UK characteristics are attributed to different regions or counties, such as people from Yorkshire being direct in their approach, and to an extent this can be applied to different cultures. We know these are generalisms and you should not apply such preconceptions to those you are working with.

You will have challenging discussions regarding health, financial situations and what is realistic. Some people prefer a direct approach, while others will find this uncomfortable. Adjust your approach accordingly, especially where someone's cultural background is one where discussion of personal or medical issues is viewed as negative, and therefore not an appropriate topic.

Ageing, health and dying

Another area of cultural difference is the approach to ageing and how changing needs are met. In the UK we have an open approach to consideration of moving to care provision when we are no longer able to manage on our own. For some the solution sits within a multi-generational household, where the needs of family members across the full age range need to be considered. In some cultures, the concept of ageing and dying in place is fundamental and will define expectations, and may require you to work to achieve this. (Chapter 9 discusses this in more general terms.)

This chapter can only begin to introduce cultural aspects you may need to consider. For us it has been an education and an opportunity to reflect on how much we don't know and need to learn, and how our practice and approach have evolved since graduation. As we write this, our focus is on ableism and educating ourselves about how stereotypes, language and unconscious bias within practice can be removed, reflecting the evolution of our profession.

9

Sensitive or Difficult Conversations

Knowledge check

* Consider your home and the room where you sleep and the bed
  you sleep in. Now think about alternative locations that provide a
  space for a bed and sleeping in a (single) hospital bed. Reviewing
  these, how many would you agree to today if we were to visit
  your home, sit down with you, and advise that your sleeping
  arrangements had to change? Being honest, probably very few
  (if any), and our discussion could be quite uncomfortable and
  emotionally charged as you digested the realization that you
  had some difficult decisions to make.

A thread running throughout this book is that our homes have meanings
to us beyond the shelter they provide. As occupational therapists working
in social care and housing, you will primarily be having conversations with
those you support when they are in their homes. Here you 'intrude' into a
personal space, and your role is to make suggestions as to how the space can
be altered or used differently.

This chapter does not aim to tell you how to have difficult conversations,
or the way to resolve a difference of opinion. Rather, it is more about considering when you might expect a challenging conversation so you can reflect
on how you think the discussion might go, and having a few suggestions
ready rather than thinking on your feet. Many of the scenarios listed will be
raised in some form throughout the book, so the questions may be here but
the answers found elsewhere!

Managing expectations

Many challenging conversations arise from raised or high expectations that are either outside of the occupational therapist's remit or exceed available budgets. For DFGs and other grant-funded work, the top line funding amount is what catches the eye, not the words before it that indicate that works are funded 'up to' this amount. This sits alongside the interpretation of any criteria, such as requesting a sensory or therapeutic space. It may be that your assessment and recommendation can achieve this, but usually not as a need in itself. Where there are two or more disabled people in a property, access to a facility such as a bathroom can be interpreted as a bathroom for the sole use of one person. In reality you will be ensuring access to a facility that could include the existing bathroom, or the creation of an additional shared space. You need to manage any expectation that an adaptation will always be an extension.

Ensuring that the right information is provided extends to professionals, as there is nothing more frustrating than being told 'X told me that I was entitled to Y'. People expect those working with them in a professional capacity to provide accurate information, but if they don't understand the criteria or what is realistic, you can be set up to start your involvement on the back foot.

Rehousing

This is more of an advisory conversation rather than the remit of an occupational therapist in social care. If you are working in a housing team, your role may include responsibility for in-depth discussions and allocation of alternative accommodation. Most social landlords will consider rehousing as part of their decision-making around meeting a tenant's needs and best use of their housing stock. Often this is written into a tenant's agreement.

It can be difficult for a person to consider moving from the place they identify strongly with, especially if it has been the family home for a significant length of time. (Consider your reflection on 'home' at the start of this book.) Your role is to ensure that tenants are aware early on in any conversations that this is something that they will be asked to consider.

If it is not part of your remit, it is appropriate to leave in-depth conversations on this topic to the tenant and relevant housing officer. While you can offer advice and information around what is needed, it is advisable to take a step back until a decision is made. You should, of course, be available for any environmental assessments of properties being considered, as you don't want to find that someone has moved to a property that requires more adaptations than the first one!

Use of rooms

We utilize rooms to suit how we live our lives. This may mean that a specific room has (in one person's opinion) a definitive label and use. Rooms that may fall into this category include:

- Second reception room.

- Dining room.

- Playroom.

- Study.

- Craft room.

- Family member's bedroom.

- Guest bedroom.

- Master bedroom.

Of course, not everyone has this wide choice of rooms in their home, and not everyone will find a suggestion to alter use difficult to adapt to. Where there is suitable space on the ground floor, it may be that you can see that a dining or second reception room is rarely used and 'kept' for family occasions or guests. Discussing how frequently these occur and alternatives to how visitors can be welcomed into other rooms in the home can lead to a realization that the space is, in fact, not used effectively.

Dining rooms can be utilized as ground floor bedrooms, but if there is no alternative space for a table and chairs (of a size to meet everyday family routines), then consider if providing a bedroom is then a barrier to mealtimes and nutrition.

Play or games rooms can be seen as essential in a busy family environment. Here, discussions have to be around what the family sees as a priority. If they decide that the playroom is essential, then your role is to manage expectations, as it is highly unlikely an adaptation would be agreed to create a new space. A study or craft room is often a place for adults to engage in meaningful leisure activities that are important to their health and wellbeing. Excluding utilizing these alternative spaces is often not a feasible option, unless the room has a financial income associated with it, such as using a study for home-based working.

Bedrooms are theoretically flexible spaces, but you would be surprised how inflexible some people can be. Parents may decline moving out of the master bedroom to a smaller double room simply because, as the adults in the household, they should have the largest bedroom space. Also, bedrooms can be designated as a guest room or space to allow for future expansion of their family. If a person's social life is home-based with frequent visitors, then there is scope for discussion with the grants or housing officer, but if it is kept 'just in case', then you need to open up the discussion. Repurposing space in a home can be like playing chess – each move is tactical, and can have unintended results.

Sensitive subjects

Health, wealth, bodily functions and death are subjects that people may find difficult to discuss openly. For health this may be because they have not understood or accepted the implications of a diagnosis or prognosis. Alternatively, it may be because those supporting them (often parents) are either in the same position or are limiting the amount of information that is provided to 'protect' them. You may find yourself having convoluted discussions, skirting round a subject that 'must not be mentioned' or meeting a blank wall of denial. You can only do your best within the parameters you are given. Where information about a diagnosis has not been given, you can discuss (away from the person) possible benefits of the person being able to make a decision with a greater understanding of their circumstances. You are then well placed to ask the question 'What is important to you?' to inform future decisions.

Mental health is affected by the barriers we face. If these are in our home, the impact can be significant. If we do not understand how someone feels, if their mood is low or variable, or if they have a mental health condition that affects cognition, how will we be able to assess whether an adaptation can support them? It may be that what you view as an insignificant barrier is the one thing that is affecting their mood. Also, are they in a position to decide at the time of asking? Someone with depression may decline a suggestion as they do not feel they 'deserve' to be helped, or they do not have the mental energy required to weigh up options.

Money (or lack of it) is not something we openly discuss with strangers, and often not with family members. Do your family members know exactly what you earn and what you spend your money on? Probably not to the detail a grant application requires. Some couples have shared bank accounts; others may have never disclosed income or savings to their partner. Children may have lasting power of attorney in financial matters; others may not even know which bank their parent uses. Lack of money can be seen as stigmatizing, and with rising costs, concern about being asked to contribute may lead to a person declining a suggested adaptation without a financial assessment.

Bodily functions are often only discussed with medical professionals or in a comedic manner (toilet humour at its most literal). In reality we are probably considering the activities of toileting and sex. Toileting (including menstruation) as a topic of conversation within an occupational therapy assessment is probably one that is expected, and up to a point accepted, but possibly not to the level of detail you may require. For children and young adults this may be excruciatingly embarrassing if the subject is raised with parents or other family members around. They may prefer for you to pose the questions in a one-to-one situation, or for them to provide answers via their parent.

You are viewed as a professional who is there to provide access to essential facilities, and people may be rather surprised that you would be raising sex as a topic for discussion. (In fact, you may be surprised that this has been included in a book about housing adaptations...) We are not, however, suggesting that your role be extended to include that of a sex therapist – far from it!

There are conversations around privacy and dignity for children as they mature into young adults; with those wanting to be intimate with their partner; and around ensuring that (in very general terms) bedroom facilities are appropriate. Do not presume that a couple in their 80s are not sexually active – this may be a key part of their relationship.

Have you considered:

- The need or preference to wash after sex?
- That profiling ('hospital') beds are usually single beds?
- The impact of suggesting someone sleeps downstairs while their partner remains upstairs?
- The need for formal carer support at set times of the day?

Do not presume that just because someone has a medical condition, is disabled or in pain that they do not have sexual needs. An uncomfortable conversation? Yes, frequently, but one you need to be open to having and able to initiate.

Family and friends

Family and friends often step in to make decisions on a person's behalf when they perceive that person is ill or frail, or in the case of children, when they consider it part of their parental role. Be sensitive to this, and ensure that you are doing all you can to hear the voice of the person you are supporting, and that their voice is heard by all involved.

Adaptations where the person's preferences are not considered will not be as successful as those that involve the person to the most appropriate extent. What do we mean by less successful? A child who is anxious about sleeping on a different floor to their parents may wake more often and ask for their parents to assist them frequently through the night. It may be that they don't need help with toileting or a drink etc., but the reassurance of seeing their parent. The outcome is that everyone's sleep is disturbed.

A person who does not enjoy the sensation of a shower is going to be more reluctant to be bathed. This may result in behaviours that challenge arising from anxiety, frustration or an inability to explain how they feel about this activity. The decisions made on their behalf may have been with the best intention, but if the person feels excluded or unable to make their voice heard, the adaptation may become a source of tension or remain unused.

End of life and life-limiting conditions

There are times where you will be supporting a person with a terminal illness, or their lifespan is foreshortened. How is that reflected in the conversations you will have around housing adaptations? First, how do you support those people with life-limiting conditions? Just because you 'know' they won't live as long as their peers, does this mean that you should limit your support to equipment? Definitely not. If we consider two conditions, muscular dystrophy and cystic fibrosis, the life expectancy for those living with these conditions has increased, where there is now an expectation they will at least mature into a young adult. Your involvement and willingness to address sensitive subjects will enable you to ask what is important to them, and from this, to improve their quality of life.

When working with people with life-limiting conditions you will need support from the multi-disciplinary team working with them to understand what is appropriate, what is likely to be needed and when. The challenge is often, when do you intervene? For someone with a diagnosis of multiple sclerosis, their presentation and prognosis may necessitate the need for extensive changes to their home environment soon after diagnosis, or their disease progression is slow, and equipment and advice suffice for a significant length of time.

Some, when hearing that they or a family member have a life-limiting condition, want 'everything' done all at once. Is this the right thing to do? Would this not run the risk of disabling rather than enabling a person? Yes, fully adapting a property will limit disruption later on, but how can you be certain that what you are recommending will, in fact, meet their long-term needs? Developing this topic further means advance care planning and planning to meet future needs. Occupational therapists' USP of balancing the medical and social model of disability will enable you to understand progression of a disease or condition. From this understanding you can project future housing needs, thus contributing to the multi-disciplinary team and support meeting expected needs as they occur.

'Where is my crystal ball', you ask? How else can you make these predictions? This is one of occupational therapy's USPs. You don't need a crystal ball; you have your assessment and activity analysis skills, your holistic approach, knowledge of both the medical and social model of disability, and an understanding of deterioration and how it limits function or engagement in occupations. To this add your ability to synthesize all of this to understand a person's situation and apply that to how they live.

For those within the last few months of their lives you need to consider their wishes and preferences as well as their health and physical presentation. Not everyone will want or need an adaptation; it may be that there are identified areas of support that are beyond equipment provision.

Ramps and rails can be added quite easily to most properties and assist as mobility declines. Where a property has limited internal access, door widening may be required to enable access to key rooms. What is more difficult to resolve is access between floors and to bathing and toileting. Stairlifts can support transfer between floors, but is a through floor lift appropriate? This is not just about money and finances. Are the building works going to be too intrusive? Can they be completed within the timescale predicted? Do not dismiss building solutions outright, but consider and discuss all aspects prior to making any recommendation.

Bathing and toileting solutions that provide and promote privacy and dignity will be a key area of provision. It is unlikely that an external brick-built bathroom adaptation will be provided within the timescale identified – even where a recommendation is prioritized. It may be that a 'pod' adaptation is possible. Shower rooms or toilets that are constructed off-site can be installed in a short space of time, although they are still subject to planning requirements.

There are times when the advice you give is not to consider adaptations. A person may be determined that this is the right action for them, but your knowledge of the processes involved means that it is unlikely that any benefit will be gained. This may be because the professionals involved in the person's end-of-life care advise that they are unlikely to live long enough to gain any benefit. An alternative scenario is that an adaptation is intended to promote independence in an occupation or activity, but the progression of a person's degenerative condition is such that they will not be able to utilize the facility.

To illustrate this, a recommendation for a ramp and powered door opener was submitted to promote independent access for a powered wheelchair user. Due to deterioration in their condition, they could no longer operate the powered wheelchair safely. A review of the recommendation identified that the powered door opener was no longer appropriate as they could not use it independently. The decision to remove this aspect highlighted the loss of independence and autonomy, and meant that the person was reluctant to accept the revision. To resolve this the discussions about the change to the scheme were difficult, touching on many aspects, and in part supported the person in their acceptance of their changing abilities.

Sensitive conversations extend beyond a person's home. Sometimes we can feel constrained by organizational boundaries. It is important to advocate and provide your professional reasoning to ensure that the right outcome is achieved. Approach discussions in a professional manner, confident that your approach is meeting a person's changing needs, maintaining an awareness of your role and theirs.

When discussing the inclusion of this chapter in the book we envisioned it would focus on rehousing and end of life. It has evolved, covering a broader range of topics. Be sensitive to the subject of any discussion and listen as much to what is not being said as to what you hear or observe. You must tread between a realistic approach promoting independence and the ability to choose, and a pragmatic approach that understands what is achievable.

10

Diverse Housing Stock

SARAH HARRIS

Knowledge check

* List as many types of domestic dwelling as you can think of.

* What is meant by 'non-standard construction'?

* What is a 'flying freehold'?

The appearance, type and construction of properties across the UK differ, providing the character we associate with different regions. Housing stock in a city meets the need of a large population within a restricted area, whereas a rural setting affords increased space. Vernacular construction reflects local building materials and weather conditions, for example buildings in the Scottish Isles typically have a low profile and small windows. Modern construction materials provide greater thermal efficiency and have increased design choices. However, this is balanced by a preference for buildings to reflect local character, and to construct building developments in the most economical method. Different buildings require different approaches to minimize the impact of restrictions afforded by their design.

This chapter identifies the most common types of dwelling within the UK, and offers brief insights into managing adaptations for these buildings.

What is a 'traditional' house?

A traditional house in the UK varies across the country, most often with brick or block wall construction, with solid or cavity walls depending on when they were built. Less frequent construction methods include metal-framed, precast concrete and in-situ concrete and timber frames.

We often refer to properties by their type, including house, 'semi', terrace, bungalow, flat, apartment, mews, caravan and houseboat, although this does not always convey sufficient detail (compare Coronation Street with The Royal Terrace in Bath, for example, both terraced streets, the former Edwardian, the latter Georgian).

Different property types present challenges to occupational therapists when planning adaptations to meet identified needs. Environmental restrictions create barriers preventing a person carrying out their activities of daily living. A pragmatic view accepts that some properties are not adaptable to meet a person's needs, but not for want of trying.

Detached house

Detached houses are standalone properties that do not share any party walls. A detached property often has its own driveway and/or a garage. Typically, it will have its own garden or outside space and land at the front, side and rear.

Semi-detached house

A semi-detached property (often called a 'semi') means that it abuts another property via a common wall. These buildings are usually designed as a mirror image of the property they are attached to. A disadvantage to a semi-detached property is sound transference; neighbours can hear sounds such as speech, doors closing, the television and music. Everyday noises are usually within personal tolerance levels, but sound transference can be particularly important if there is an autistic person in the household. For example, the location of their bedroom in relation to the party wall can influence this, both in relation to their noise sensitivity and potentially increased volume or repetitive noise, affecting neighbours.

Terraced house

A terraced house may be a mid-terrace or an end-of-terrace property, the length of a terrace varying depending on location. Usually, they are a row of houses, but can be built around a courtyard. Row houses are single-storey terraces, and mews houses are similar, but converted from stables and garages.

Some terraces do not have a front garden and lead directly on to the public highway or pavement. The public highway is communal, meaning you cannot provide a ramp or step-lift. Some have small front gardens, which means that there isn't always scope to construct a ramp, and a step-lift is the only option at the front access.

Access to terraced houses may be via a shared passage, with front doors for adjoining properties placed partway down the passage. This does not provide space for wheelchair access into the property. To the rear may be a yard (concrete, flagged or a grass area); this can be landlocked, which means there is no access beyond the property to get out of this space. Some terraced properties have access to a rear communal alleyway – where the surface finish could be uneven or poorly maintained, and access points may not be kept clear, making them inaccessible.

Some properties have two reception rooms downstairs (parlours) – one is a living room and the other one may be a dining room or utilized as a bedroom. Consideration must be taken when using one room as a bedroom because, depending on the configuration, one room may lead to the kitchen, so cannot be used as a bedroom. If using one living room as a bedroom, consider how the person is going to access bathing, which could be on a different floor.

A challenge with adapting terraced properties is that the stairs are often steep and narrow. There may be a small landing with a further step up to first floor rooms on either side. The foot of the stairs may be located directly in front of the front door. In addition to steps at the top of the stairs, there may be single steps at the entrance to rooms at the rear of the house.

Some terraces have a ground floor bathroom situated at the end of the property off the kitchen, with no bathing or toileting facilities upstairs. Using the toilet at night would require the person to negotiate the stairs and then travel through the property.

Maisonette

These are typically described as a two-storey property with its own entrance. You can think of them as a house that is over a flat, or two houses, one on top of another. They may be over shops and then the stairs are likely to be external. External stairs may be concrete, poorly lit and for some add to concerns about their personal safety. Some have metal gates installed at the base for security, but don't always have an intercom, making reaching the gate difficult for a person with disabilities. Some maisonettes may be over a garage (which is not always owned by the person living in the maisonette), and don't always have an outdoor space. The top maisonette often has communal stairs, making it unlikely a stair or platform lift can be installed. Remember that in a maisonette there are internal stairs (just like a house).

Town house

This is a terraced or semi-detached property, with living space on three or more floors. This design is increasingly common in new developments. Some older properties of this type are prefabricated (prefab) constructions built as temporary accommodation after 1945, and remain occupied. They may have had cladding fitted to update them, so their appearance is of a more robust construction, although the fabric has not been altered.

A typical town house has three floors: a ground floor entrance, living room (or bedroom), toilet and kitchen. The first floor has bedrooms and the family bathroom; the third floor the master bedroom and an en suite. The first floor bathroom may consist of a bath and wash hand basin, and the toilet can be across the landing, in a separate room. A benefit of this layout is there is often scope for ground floor living, but in properties where the main living room is on the first floor, this is likely to limit family interaction. As the largest bedroom is typically on the top floor, it may be a challenge to install through floor lifts or even stairlifts.

Bungalow

This is usually a single-storey dwelling. Dormer bungalows have a second storey, often with steeply pitched ceilings. Historically, bungalows built as retirement homes or social housing for those over a set age are not always accessible – they can have small interior proportions, and no space for wheelchair turning circles, offering limited scope for adaptations. Typically, they will have two bedrooms. Some bungalows of this type have small second bedrooms, and this may be difficult if the moving group is three adults – a couple and an adult with a disability, for example. The second bedroom does not always have sufficient space for a wheelchair user.

Housing associations often restrict the age group of these types of properties to those 50+ years old, requiring everyone in the household to be over this age. This means that the property may meet a disabled child's assessed needs, but the age policy prevents the parent taking on the tenancy.

Social housing developments of bungalows may have communal

gardens, which may be an issue for installing ramps. Where a landlord owns a property, they may not accept pets, which is a challenge for those who are downsizing. If pets are allowed, communal gardens can be an issue because there is no enclosed garden to keep the pet (typically a dog) within a defined area.

Many bungalows have a step at the front door and a porch that is not wheelchair accessible. Rear doors providing garden access may be directly off the kitchen; while most doors in the property are 726mm wide, the rear door may have a reduced width.

Older bungalows often sit on larger plots, which can offer scope for extensions, and some new-build bungalows are designed to be spacious and are wheelchair accessible, with level front and rear access.

Flats and bedsits

Flats or similar properties are often rented or leasehold, so it is essential to make sure you are aware of the tenure and any restrictions before recommending an adaptation. Flats or apartments (they are the same thing, but developers use 'apartment', as it sounds more luxurious!) may be in purpose-built units or blocks, above business premises or a conversion of an existing building.

Cottage (or four-in-a-block) flats provide ground floor or first floor living with individual entrances. The ground floor may be difficult to adapt for a wheelchair user due to supporting walls. Often bathrooms have a separate toilet, with neither room offering sufficient space for a wheelchair user. It may be possible to take space from an adjacent room to increase the bathroom size, or combine the bathroom and toilet.

Flats may be multi-storey or high-rise, with or without lift access. Walk-up flats have communal entrances; fire regulations mean they can have a heavy communal door (often not automated), which is linked to an intercom system and not always adaptable. There can be internal steps to ground floor flats and external steps to access outdoor space.

Bedsits are flats where the lounge and bedroom are one room, with a separate kitchen and bathroom. Studio flats have an open kitchen area and sleeping and living space. They are generally small, not wheelchair accessible and without scope to increase space.

House conversions use large properties to create flats, which can be any variety of layouts. This includes basements, often with external steps down or an external ramp to the access point.

Flats may be within purpose-built extra-care schemes that have lifts, caregivers on site and a receptionist. However, don't presume that because this is specialist provision it will meet everyone's needs. Access is usually level and they generally have wheelchair-accessible bathrooms (but not all), and often wet rooms. Doors can be an issue due to a need for fire doors and, depending on how access to the door is achieved (usually via a fob), any powered door opener must link to the internal fob system, which may also be an issue.

High-rise or tower blocks

These are a challenge to adapt due to the complex construction and location of services. Older buildings may not have a lift installed. Some landlords have policies about letting this type of accommodation to people with disabilities, due to concerns over emergency egress in a fire (there needs to be an evacuation plan). Floor design often prevents installation of a level-access shower. There may be space for a shower tray with a ramp, but these do not suit all wheelchair users, especially as bathrooms tend to be small. Many shower trays need an electric pump to boost removal of grey water.[1]

Static caravan, mobile home, park home or lodge

All four of these names refer to the same provision. They all are prefabricated homes with the potential to be resited. They are usually sited within a park, and often the unit itself is owned but the ground is leased. There may be restrictions on any external changes as part of the lease agreement, and leases may have a clause stating that the property must be vacated for a set period, in line with a site's planning permission.

While it is possible to adapt them, the construction is likely to require strengthening to allow for floor, wall or ceiling fixed equipment. The installation at a site means that these are not level access, so a ramp or platform lift will be required for wheelchair users.

Houseboat, narrowboat or barge

These are boats that have been designed or modified to be used as dwellings. They are usually motorized and tend to be moored or kept stationary at a set location, and are often tethered to land utilities. Some can be adapted to

---

1   Grey water is from the shower, bath or basin. Black wastewater refers to water from the toilet.

be wheelchair accessible, but you will need support from a marine engineer as this is a highly specialized area and, like buildings, must conform to set regulations.

Non-standard construction

Typically, properties in the UK are constructed of brick or stone with a slate or tile roof. When thinking about non-standard construction, start by imagining a thatched cottage – very clearly not your typical construction. Not all are so obvious. Some houses are 'mud and stud'/cob/wattle and daub construction, but when covered in a lime render appear to be brick or block built. Some prefab buildings have now been faced with brick, so appearances may be deceptive!

Non-standard construction doesn't just relate to heritage or older properties.[2] It can include:

- Steel or timber frames.

- Prefabricated or modular.

- Concrete.

- Straw.

Self-build projects may utilize non-standard construction techniques, so this is not just an issue associated with older properties – just look at a few episodes of the Channel 4 television programme *Grand Designs*! The challenge with many forms of non-standard construction is that they may not be sufficiently robust to facilitate the addition of wall-mounted equipment, such as changing benches or even grab rails or a tracked hoist system, due to the construction of the upper floors or walls.

Garage conversions

Garages are rarely used for vehicles these days; therefore, they are often identified as usable space for adaptations. Garages are not always connected to the main property – they may be adjacent to a side wall or integrated. They are not always suitable for adapting, and challenges include (in no particular order):

---

2   Non Standard House Construction provides some information and highlights some designs where the ground floor construction differs from the upper floors: https://nonstandardhouse.com/various-houses-of-non-traditional-construction

- A different floor height to the main building.

- They may be single-skin construction.

- They may have a flat roof (so are not suitable if someone needs hoisting).

- They don't always have utilities installed.

- Access may be via the staircase in the main part of the house, preventing door widening.

- Single garages may not provide sufficient width for equipment and access once insulated.

On a positive note:

- Garages are often 'free' space, maintaining current room usage.

- The garage door can be converted into a window and door.

- New-builds often have garages adjacent to the ground toilet and/or utility room, providing access to water and waste.

Conversion of outbuildings

Like garages, these are normally single-skin dwellings, and they need to have a double-skin construction to be considered as a habitable dwelling, although increasing the thickness of the wall usually results in reduced internal space.

Some homes have an outside toilet (which is cold in the winter and hot in the summer) adjacent to a coal shed. These often appear to provide additional space but are not always attached to the property or suitable for adapting. The cost of converting these often exceeds building an extension to provide the same end result.

Listed buildings and conservation areas

A listed building is one that has been placed on one of the four statutory lists maintained by Historic England, Historic Environment Scotland, Cadw in Wales, or the Northern Ireland Environment Agency. The specific listing will have implications for adaptations with restrictions on changes you can make to a listed building without permission. Some buildings may only have their exterior listed, while for others the listing includes the internal structure and appearance. Listed building status helps to protect them from demolition, and ensures that future generations will still get a chance to appreciate their beauty and historical significance.

New-build

New-build properties can be interpreted as still within their 10-year guarantee period.

Guidance is in place for wheelchair-accessible properties, but not all are built to this standard. New-builds tend to be built with level access to the property (typically at both the front and rear), widened doors and a toilet on the ground floor, although this does not automatically mean they are fully accessible.

A note of caution: There is often a difference between plot numbers and the allocated house number. If you are referring to online planning documents, you will need to ensure you are referring to the correct property!

Porches

Porches provide shelter, but also present barriers to access. Many houses have a porch that can be difficult to adapt due to split floor levels and thresholds. The threshold could be a combination frame, which is a door and a window frame, so changing the door may require changing the full door and window set. The door configuration can also be an issue. Some have one door that opens inwards or one door that opens out; some have a split door; and some have a double patio door. Porches are also used as storage areas or boot rooms, reducing ease of access.

Flying freehold and party walls

'Flying freehold' is a legal term describing part of a property that overhangs a neighbouring property or plot. Examples include first floor rooms over a passageway or driveway (a semi-detached or terraced property) or a balcony extending outside of the curtilage of a plot.

'Party walls' are shared walls either between two (or more) dwellings, or where a wall forms part of a boundary between two plots. Where adaptations are proposed there is a legal requirement for permission to be gained from all parties involved.

This is only a whistle-stop tour to demonstrate the variety of properties found in the built environment. It is not exhaustive, offering only brief guidance on some aspects of adapting a property type. The advice is to ask questions (and keep asking questions), and with experience, you will be able to predict pitfalls and plan adaptations with confidence.

11

Adaptations for Children and Young People

```
┌ ─ ─ ─ ─ ─ ─ ─ ─ ─ ─ ─ ─ ─ ─ ─ ─ ─ ─ ─ ─ ─ ─ ─ ─ ─ ─ ─ ─ ─ ─ ┐
```

Knowledge check

*   How do children's key occupations differ from those of adults?

*   What is meant by 'age and stage'?

*   What different methods can you use to communicate the concept of an adaptation to a child?

```
└ ─ ─ ─ ─ ─ ─ ─ ─ ─ ─ ─ ─ ─ ─ ─ ─ ─ ─ ─ ─ ─ ─ ─ ─ ─ ─ ─ ─ ─ ─ ┘
```

Let's think about who we mean by a 'child' or 'young person'. In simple terms, it is bracketed by an age range: 0 to 18 years. Well, that's the easy bit over and done with, except that not all teams will use this definition. An integrated team might adopt 19, mirroring the age range in special school provision, or alternatively adopt the approach of special education and disability (SEND), which extends to 25.

One way or another, this is a population with a unique characteristic – the degree of change must be taken into account. Consider the differences between a toddler and a 10-year-old, and that is without the need to factor in the impact of a health condition or disability.

Before you begin to think this is going to be complicated and not for you, let's go back to basics. First, your secret weapon: the occupational therapy process remains exactly the same whether you are working with a child or an adult. Second, your understanding of meaningful occupations: consider a 24-hour period – we all sleep, eat, manage our personal care, complete some form of work and (hopefully) have leisure time. The main difference is terminology – exchange 'education' for 'work' and 'play' for 'leisure' and there is no difference between an adult's and a child's day. Those with health conditions or disabilities will need to engage with these occupations whatever their age.

So why is there a need for a chapter on this when there is information in the rest of the book to support you? Yes, much of the information elsewhere in the book will be relevant, but in this chapter the focus is on what you will be considering as you plan the most appropriate way to meet identified needs for children and young people. While most using this book will be based in social care or housing and working within the social model of disability, you need to transfer across to the medical model and consider the implications of a diagnosis or a condition. Consider this alongside any identified needs at the time of your assessment, and how you can minimize the impact of these now, and through to adulthood.

Broadly speaking, commonly seen conditions or diagnoses can be divided into three categories: those that are evident at or soon after birth; those that become apparent over time; and those arising from an unexpected incident or illness. Cerebral palsy and spina bifida are examples when the likelihood a child may have additional needs is identified at an early age. Global developmental delay is when a child takes longer to achieve key developmental milestones such as speech, learning to walk or social interactions skills. This, and conditions such as muscular dystrophy or spinal muscular atrophy, usually become apparent as a child does not reach expected milestones or a change in their abilities is identified. Illness or an accident can result in a disability in an otherwise healthy child or young person. Incidence in the total population is low, but meningitis, encephalitis or a significant injury can result in a long-term or permanent impairment. As we can't provide an extensive list of conditions you may encounter when working with children here, the internet and your preferred search engine will be your best source of information!

You will be working with children and young people through to adulthood. Some you will meet at a young age, providing opportunities to develop long-term relationships, working with them and their families to adapt to their changing needs. Others you will meet at the point they have experienced an unexpected event, a diagnosis, illness or accident, where the expectations of what life looks like to them, and their family, will have changed.

Resilience and acceptance vary from person to person and family to family. Just because a diagnosis has been given at an early age does not mean that the family have been able to adjust to and accept this news.

Conversely, a child, young person or family may be more resilient than you expect, following an unexpected change in abilities or needs.

Conversations and the voice of the child

You will be having conversations with a wide range of adults including parents, medical professionals, grants officers, surveyors and contractors. At the centre of everything you are aiming to achieve is the child or young person you are working with. While it is paramount that they are part of the conversation as far as possible, limiting factors to this may not just be due to their ability to communicate or cognitive ability. Parents may wish to limit the amount of information a child is given about their condition or prognosis, making it tricky to plan for the long term – it is difficult to discuss a bedroom layout to enable hoist transfers or a bathroom with a shower bench if the child or young person isn't aware that they will eventually need this level of support. Some may not want to have this type of conversation, and just want you to tell them what you recommend. Think back to the 'ladder of participation' (or, if you have jumped straight in here, have a look at Chapter 3). You may need to adjust your approach to actively involve them in any decision-making.

Concepts such as changing the layout of a room or building an extension may be difficult to grasp, so use any methods that might help. Photos, drawings, marking out the space on the floor and even LEGO® models may help in explaining what outcomes you are aiming for. All we can say is work within the parameters you have, and wherever possible involve the child or young person – and don't forget to record their voice in your case notes!

Meeting the need for adaptations

The adaptation criteria within the DFG provide a way of highlighting the different areas you will be addressing. As mentioned previously we all have the same meaningful occupations, but it is highly unlikely that you will be recommending adaptations to support a child or young person's access to home-based employment or as a caregiver – but never say never.

Rather than list each of the areas of occupation, let's think about how a child or young person differs from an adult in regard to meeting needs through adaptations.

Change (or development) and growth happens to us all. Sometimes the direction is progression, and sometimes regression, meaning both skill acquisition and loss need to be accommodated. Most children will become teenagers and then young adults. However, do not limit yourself and your recommendations based on a prognosis or timescale. Sadly, not all children live to adulthood, but there are many occasions where a child with a life-limiting condition lives beyond their predicted life span. Therefore, you should be planning for long-term needs rather than limiting your focus to immediate needs. This is one of those times where there is no set answer, and decision-making will be a balance between practicality and a positive approach.

Allowing for change and development

A challenge to be considered is size. You cannot and should not plan an adaptation around the size a child is now, otherwise you will be constantly revisiting and revising provision, which will not be popular with those involved. It may be difficult for parents looking at a toddler to appreciate that you need to be planning for when they are 16. This forward planning may appear unnecessary when you are recommending a room size that allows for adult-sized equipment such as a profiling bed while their child is still in a cot, or if you are ensuring space is available for a through floor lift where the hope is that the child will become mobile.

Ideally this forward planning will include the structural changes needed to facilitate future provision of equipment, for example, including noggins to strengthen ceilings and joists for a ceiling track hoist, and fused spurs for charge points or power supply for hoists, adjustable height-changing benches and wash and dry toilets etc.

How you consider development and actions can be based around 'age and stage'. What is appropriate for that child or young person, and what stage of development have they achieved? These may be not in line with typical development, and so a person-centred approach is essential as you are adapting a property to meet their needs rather than the needs of a typically developing person.

Bathing and toileting are areas where growth and development present some challenges, particularly if parental expectations don't align with what has been proposed. Two frequent topics for discussion are a bath for young children and a ground floor toilet to support a toileting programme.

First, bathing: parents' expectations are often that young children will enjoy a 'traditional' bath routine, which later changes to a shower for older children. The wording of the DFG criteria does not exclude access to both a bath and a shower, although this may not be practical within the space available and within the financial limits. This can be a difficult discussion, especially if there are younger siblings, who, in the parents' view, will miss out on a key part of childhood.

Then, a wish for a child to become continent, even if not fully independent in toileting, is an understandable aim. However, the provision of an additional toilet to support the introduction of a toileting programme is not appropriate without a realistic expectation that the child will become continent. It is a tricky conundrum as lack of access to a toilet may be the factor preventing this skill being developed. While each situation needs to be considered on merit, you should ensure that at least one existing toilet is accessible, and that additional information from other professionals has been accessed to assist in your decision-making.

Privacy and dignity

Development and maturity usually bring independence, especially in personal or intimate care. Where a teenager or young adult hasn't achieved the ability to manage this without assistance, try to enable this area of provision to be completed in the most appropriate way. Sometimes parents will continue to meet a need in the same way that they did when their child was much younger – perhaps changing incontinence products in a family space, just as you might do for a toddler (here we accept that everyone will have their own opinion of if this is appropriate for a baby or toddler...). This can be one of the more difficult conversations to initiate, as they may not appreciate your point of view. You should be enabling and encouraging these activities to be completed with privacy and dignity, such as ensuring that if a caregiver needs to remain in a room while someone uses the toilet, then the door can be fully closed. If a child or young person has sitting balance but cannot manage their personal care after toileting, then a conversation about installing a wash and dry toilet is appropriate, even if they aren't continent.

Mobility

Mobility is something that is developed over time and may be a delayed milestone. A mobility aid might be required for the child or young person to achieve independence, or it may be that your planning is based around an expectation the child will become a full-time wheelchair user.

If you are thinking about wheelchair use, consider if the child or young person will self-propel, need assistance or use a powered wheelchair.

The decision-making around this will be supported by information from other professionals including physiotherapists and the wheelchair provider. Your decisions won't just be around ramps and door widening; they will include the location of facilities – is ground floor living required, for instance? It is tricky to accurately predict development in this area, especially if the adaptation is completed while the child is young. Do the risks associated with carrying a child up and down stairs outweigh adopting a wait and see approach?

Cognition

A child's cognitive ability is another area of development that will guide adaptation planning. This is difficult to predict, especially where there is limited communication ability, or the child is at a stage of development where abstract concepts or potential situations cannot be understood. It may be that you plan for later adaptations, such as ensuring that a scheme allows for a door opener to be installed at a later date, rather than presume that this will not be required. Understanding if a child or young person has capacity is a key factor – not only when considering if a **restrictive practice** is in place, but also in all interactions, ensuring a child's voice is heard.

Household structure

Families come in all shapes and sizes, but one thing is certain when planning a home adaptation for a child or young person – they will have a family, even if they are not related by birth. This means that your assessment and recommendations will need to be holistic, considering the needs of all family members. This may mean that there are others who need specialist provision, either through your involvement or through joint working with another team, so embrace the opportunity to collaborate if it arises.

Most discussions will involve the parents and the child or young person you are supporting, but it may be that others need to be involved in the decision-making. Who has which bedroom can be a difficult decision for a sibling who is asked to vacate 'their' space. Some families will want to discuss this among themselves, while others may take an approach that this should be part of the discussions you are having. Yet again, there is no definitive answer to this.

Families are fluid – older siblings may leave the home (and in some cases, return), younger siblings may be born. Obviously, each family has the right to decide how they live and plan their lives, but basing plans on an older sibling leaving home has two disadvantages. First, this delays meeting identified needs, and second, what if they decide they don't want to leave home? Planning around younger siblings can only take place if they have been born. This may seem a bit of an odd comment when families may have a clear plan to have x number of children. You cannot ask for an additional bedroom for the child you are supporting if there are unused bedrooms available for you to work with. Having an early conversation around working within the existing structure of the property may help with this, but it may seem unfair to parents that you are not working within their life plans and expectations.

Complex medical needs

Advances in medical science, and parental expectations that children with complex medical needs will live in the family home, mean that you need to take into consideration a wide range of factors. This is a population who may have a wide range of medical equipment and significant care needs, including support from formal caregivers. For instance, current DFG guidance does not specify storage of medical supplies within its criteria. The volume of incontinence products in a single delivery plus essential medical equipment can mean that a typical bedroom lacks sufficient space. Where there are younger siblings or medications that must be kept securely, there may be a need for locked storage. Here a solution could be to use safety as your rationale. Another area of need that is not explicitly included in the DFG criteria is space for waking caregivers. As more children and young people with complex conditions are living longer and are supported in the family home, this is a need that has to be catered for. Be proactive, positive and apply your lateral thinking skills, but if you don't ask, you won't know if you can address this area of need.

Where does all this leave you? Hopefully not too daunted, and if you feel that providing adaptations for children and young people is a bit like guess work/ gazing into a crystal ball/holding a finger up to see which way the wind is blowing, then think again. (If that is the case, head straight to Chapter 5 on professional reasoning and re/read it!)

Yes, in this area of practice there are challenges, and the current financial situation is that complex adaptations may be needed but available funding does not cover the costs. Often recommendations for adaptations for children seek to resolve multiple issues. This may take longer to identify a scheme that works, and you may have to prioritize one need over another to achieve the best result you can. If you think that this could be overwhelming, indulge us for a moment as we consider an analogy.

Think of building solutions in terms of horses, zebras and unicorns – bear with us...!

Horses can be found pretty much everywhere; it doesn't take too much effort to identify where you could go and see one.

Zebras take a bit more effort. You are going to be looking for a zoo or wildlife park as (unlike llamas and alpacas) they don't appear to be found in our countryside.

Unicorns – there's no chance of seeing one of these however hard you look.

So, for building solutions, there will be many cases where the solution to an issue is pretty obvious (horses) and others where you are going to be scratching your head quite a bit, but in the end, a suitable solution can be found (zebras). And then there are situations where there isn't a practical solution at all. These are unicorns, and you may find families will be asking (hoping or expecting) you to pull this one out of the bag. Although you are working to find the best solution to a problem, be aware when you stray into looking for something that does not exist.

It doesn't have to be a request that is unreasonable. A parent asking for a bath to allow her four-year-old and baby to enjoy bath time together is not such an unusual thing. However, the bath support needed for the four-year-old does not leave any space in the bath for the baby. The request to identify a bath long enough to accommodate shared bath times is a 'unicorn'. Time spent researching extra-long baths is not time well spent, as both children will grow and the bath support will get longer. It is tough to have to say no at times, but be realistic.

Working with families in their home environment making practical changes that have a significant impact is rewarding. You are adjusting the environment that children and young people spend the majority of their time in. The work is varied, and the range of diagnoses means that you can't be a specialist in one area, but what you can be is true to your occupational therapy roots. You can utilize your core occupational therapy skills of assessment and activity analysis to truly understand how families are living their lives, applying your professional reasoning and experience (or, if you are new to this area of practice, tapping into the experience of those you are working with) to identify appropriate solutions to the issues you have identified.

This is an area of practice where you get to know the families you work with, spend time with them as the adaptation process is followed, and at the end of it, see the changes that are as a result of your actions and recommendations. In addition, you will work with a diverse team across health, social care and housing, often working as the key communicator between all the different professionals. You will bring together key pieces of information, synthesize them, and from this ensure that the adaptations meet the identified areas of need in the most effective way possible.

This chapter has offered an alternative approach to highlight key aspects of working with children, young people and their families. It is designed to be read in conjunction with other relevant chapters, supporting your decision-making to meet their long-term needs.

12

Adapting for Sensory Impairment

Knowledge check

* How many senses do we have?

* What can cause an inability to regulate body temperature?

* What is photophobia?

* What is lumen a measure of?

* How do soft furnishings affect a person's ability to hear?

Generally speaking, when people think about housing adaptations they think of big changes – ramps, level-access showers, extensions and the like. When considering adaptations to address sensory needs, the effect of 'small' changes or decisions will have a significant impact.

What do we mean by 'sensory impairment', and who should we be considering changes for? We are aware of the five senses (touch, taste, sight, sound and hearing), but there are more that we should consider, including the ability to sense temperature, proprioception (awareness of body in space) and the vestibular system (balance). While there are various schools of thought on this topic, we won't go into details here, and focus instead on sight and hearing, but we begin this chapter looking at heating and temperature regulation.

Heating and temperature regulation

The ability to regulate temperature can be affected by illness or a medical condition or because of the ageing process. Hypothyroidism and Parkinson's disease can affect the body's ability to regulate temperature. Medications may affect temperature regulation, including some antidepressants, antipsychotics and opiate pain medications. Part of our body's ability to maintain temperature is through movement, so any condition that reduces the amount a person moves may result in an increased risk of hypothermia.

Hyperthermia is usually considered an issue related to the summer months – especially as in the UK we are not that good at adapting our routines to minimize the impact of high temperatures. However, during winter, it may be that the room temperature is raised significantly, which can combine with a lack of mobility and ventilation to act on the person's body temperature. Also, some medications act on the central nervous system, which may increase temperature, and it can be a rare side effect of a brain injury.

What does this mean in the context of adaptations? It can be the simple steps, such as making sure that the person can open and close curtains, windows or doors. Can they reach them, and operate the handles or stays? Should you be investigating powered systems and linking in with smart technology to increase flexibility for temperature control?

The type of heating installed will affect the level of temperature regulation within a property. Wood or coal heating systems result in changes of temperature over a 24-hour period and require monitoring to ensure that they remain alight. Night storage heaters, which are less common these days, may be installed, although older versions may not have the flexibility to adjust when heat is released, or may not retain sufficient heat to maintain temperatures through the day and evening.

In some instances, it may be appropriate to change the heating system altogether, but this may fall outside of the adaptation remit. In this case you should signpost people to sources of support, and for tenants, provide written support for the change. One recommendation for any change to a heating system is that it should come with a portable thermostat that can be moved from room to room. This is not only sensible for those who need to ensure that they manage their temperature regulation; it also means that the heating in a property is only used where and when it is needed which, at the time of writing, is essential due to spiralling energy costs.

Moving on, we shall now look at the two 'main' senses compensated for when adapting properties: sight and hearing. These will affect all of us to an extent at some point in life, so some suggestions will have relevance even if someone does not have a formal diagnosis of vision or hearing impairment. Please remember that an impairment to one of these senses does not automatically mean that the other sense is impaired – and vice versa. This goes back to your holistic and person-centred approach and your initial assessment. For people who have both vision and hearing loss, seek specialist support from professionals working with them as they will know how best to minimize the impact of being deafblind.

Visual impairment or loss

What this means to each of us will differ, as will our ability to adapt to a change. It may be that the visual impairment has been present since birth, because of ageing or a medical condition, or as a result of trauma. Each of these will require a different approach, as will the type of visual impairment. A person can be registered blind but retain some vision, so do not take that information to mean that they have no sight at all.

Visual impairment may affect sight or the range of vision in several ways, including:

- *Loss of central vision:* This means that peripheral vision remains, but central vision is either blurred or occluded.

- *Loss of peripheral (side) vision:* This reduces or removes the clarity of the visual field outside of the central field, that is, tunnel vision.

- *Blurred vision:* Loss of acuity to the whole visual field.

- *Light sensitivity (photophobia):* Light levels can cause pain or discomfort.

- *Night blindness:* An inability to see in low light levels, or associated with difficulty in adapting to changes in light levels.

The adaptations required will depend on the circumstances of the person you are supporting, who may also need support and advice from medical professionals or specialist organizations or charities. A list of some of these is included at the end of this chapter, and other or more local sources can also be found through an internet search.

Light levels

When sunlight is strong, we wear sunglasses or a hat with a brim to assist with our vision; as light levels reduce during cloudy days or the evening, we switch lights on. If a person's visual impairment is affected by lighting, adjusting how a room is lit can be achieved by changing the type of light bulb and checking its lumen rating (the level of visible light emitted). Higher lumen ratings provide more visible light. It is also possible to select the type of light – warm or cool white – which may be more comfortable for the person.

The amount and strength of illumination achieved will depend on the size of the room and where the bulb(s) are positioned. Before confirming a lighting scheme, try out different options or positions, if possible. Is a pendant light fitting the most appropriate, or should wall lights supplement this? Standard or table lamps offer flexibility, but only if power sockets are situated in the right areas. These days there need to be sufficient power sockets to allow the use of standard or table lamps alongside all the gadgets we use daily.

If external light sources are an issue, applying glare reduction film to windows or ensuring blinds or curtains can be closed will reduce glare.

> Glare (or intrusive levels of light) doesn't always result from natural light. If a ground level room faces a busy road junction, the impact on light levels from headlights as vehicles approach and then turn may at least be a distraction, but at worst may significantly affect what can be seen.

Task lighting

Task lighting provides support in several ways, but in the context of visual impairment it is used to highlight the location where an activity takes place (e.g., over a basin for hand washing), and also to provide the specific light level or direction for that occupation.

Wayfinding

Light can be used to assist in directing people around their home. This could be leading to the entrance(s) by illuminating the route, highlighting hazards such as steps and through task lighting promoting operation of the lock. Within the home lighting can either highlight an endpoint or doorway, or alternatively low-level LED strip lighting can highlight a route. Don't discount everyday solutions either – something as low-tech as a night light or two may be all that is required.

Surface finishes

Our homes are filled with different surface finishes that affect light levels. How we decorate our spaces differs alongside the purpose of a room. Often kitchens and bathrooms have shiny surface finishes such as tiles and on cabinets (see Figure 9). This makes for easy cleaning but light 'bounces' off these surfaces, reflecting in all directions, creating glare and affecting vision. Also gloss and silk paint or metallic finishes on wallpapers contribute to this.

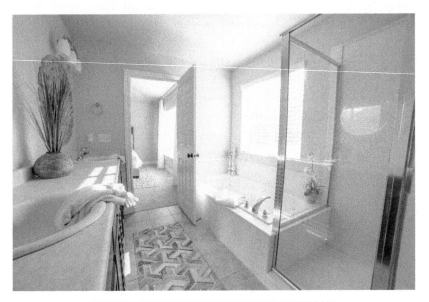

FIGURE 9. REFLECTIVE SURFACES IN THE BATHROOM

Selecting matt or low sheen finishes will reduce the impact of glare, especially when you consider the amount of surface area walls have within a home.

Colour

Considering paint finishes leads us to colour choice – a very personal choice, but one that can be used to highlight and define. The overall colour scheme should reflect the light levels tolerated by a person using tonal contrast (see Figures 15a and 15b in Chapter 14). Light, bright rooms will work for some while a much darker, muted scheme will support those who have light sensitivity.

This goes beyond paint choice and can include soft furnishings. As you are working in someone's home, however, you can advise and inform, but at the end of the day, this is often how a place is made to feel like 'home'.

Colour is useful to provide definition such as using a contrasting colour on skirting boards and architraves to define the edges of a room and doorways. It can be incorporated into wayfinding, providing a route, highlighting a change of room or through zoning to define an activity.

Controls and switches

Think about how you locate a light switch in the dark. Often low-level light outside from streetlights will assist you, but it isn't as easy as during the day. Consider white light switches on a white wall or white pull cords in a white bathroom. Switches can be highlighted through colour contrast: a band painted around them or the whole wall in a contrasting colour – or by changing the 'traditional' white switch to one that contrasts – simple solutions that apply to power sockets as well.

Pull cord switches are more challenging to locate and identify, especially if the initial attempt to locate it causes it to swing. Adding a contrasting, heavier light pull assists, as does ensuring the pull cord is at an appropriate length for the person to use. It may be that changing it to a wall switch is required.

Home safety

Assistive technology was a specialist area of provision, but now smart tech for our homes can be readily accessed, and 'high street' solutions are widely available, from timers to sensors to smart light bulbs. It may be that the adaptations you recommend are universal or 'low key', but this shouldn't diminish the impact they can have. This includes home safety, where smoke, heat and carbon monoxide detectors can be hard-wired to reduce the need to change batteries or rely on others to assist with this. Advice and information on this is available from the local Fire and Rescue Service, which often has schemes to support installation.

Another aspect of home safety is the ability to control access to our homes. Intercom systems are widely available and can be audio only as well as video, and can be controlled via apps or viewed on computer or television screens.

Hearing impairment or loss

Like vision impairment, loss or partial loss of hearing often results from the ageing process, but has many causes, and people will adjust to varying degrees, as will those around them. There is a wide variation in the ability to hear tone and volume, and the impact of tinnitus should not be forgotten.

One thing that the COVID-19 pandemic highlighted was the importance of lipreading to a far wider population – masks impact not only on the ability to read lips but also, to a certain extent, on interpreting meaning or intent through facial expressions. Ensuring that during your conversations you are facing the person and your face is not in shadow will support them to participate in discussions and understand suggestions.

Noise levels

External noise is not something we have any control over, although it is something we can consider if we are supporting someone with hearing impairment to be rehoused. The amount of external noise can be reduced using curtains or blinds, but these can't be used throughout the day, so it may be appropriate to consider the glazing in key rooms. Triple glazing will decrease the amount of sound, but only if windows can be kept closed, which is a challenge in hot weather and when keeping a room aired, such as during the pandemic. Other sources of external noise include those from lifts or escalators within blocks of flats or apartments, and from extractor fans and air conditioning systems.

Within a property noise levels can usually be controlled, but consider the impact of background noises that you probably 'tune out'. Extractor fans in the kitchen and bathroom have varying levels of decibels and can 'over run' after they are switched off. Other sources of noise within the kitchen are from fan ovens, washing machines, tumble dryers, fridges and freezers.

The surface finishes we choose as part of our décor have an effect. Compare the amount of 'echo' within your bathroom to that in your living room. The smooth surface finishes on the walls and floor of a bathroom are practical when it comes to cleaning and appropriate for that room, but they do little to 'dampen' the volume of noise as the room is used. The use of carpets and soft furnishings in a living room absorbs some of the noise, reducing the volume and echo. Where a property has hard floor surfaces the sound generated by shoes can be intrusive but could be reduced by asking visitors to remove their footwear or through the use of rugs (when they are not a trip hazard).

Home safety

We all want to remain safe within our homes, so systems that alert via flashing lights can be installed for heat, smoke and CO_2, and can be linked to apps and wearable tech. This also applies to doorbells and entry systems, to retain control over who is invited into our homes.

Not all changes require adaptations; ensuring those who wear hearing aids are supported can include low-tech solutions such as ensuring the television is located where the screen can be viewed at all times of the day and enabling the use of subtitles and visual cues. It is also possible to install hearing loops that link to hearing aids.

As professionals working with a wide range of people, you cannot be expected to know or even retain all the knowledge required to address the issues identified in your assessments. Seeking help outside of the team you are working with is not a sign that you are not competent – more that you have an awareness of your strengths and understand the importance and benefits of collaborative working. To support you in this, here are some links to charities and resources that you may find helpful when adapting for sensory impairments. Support is also available from local or regional charities and support groups.

Useful resources

Deafblind UK: https://deafblind.org.uk

Guide Dogs: www.guidedogs.org.uk

Hearing Dogs for Deaf People: www.hearingdogs.org.uk

Hearing Link Services: www.hearinglink.org

National Association of Deafened People: www.nadp.org.uk

National Deaf Children's Society: www.ndcs.org.uk/information-and-support

RNIB (Royal National Institute for Blind People): www.rnib.org.uk

Royal National Institute for Deaf People: https://rnid.org.uk

Sense: www.sense.org.uk

The Partially Sighted Society: www.partsight.org.uk

Thomas Pocklington Trust: www.pocklington-trust.org.uk

13

Supporting People with Degenerative Conditions

```
Knowledge check

*   List four degenerative conditions.

*   How many of these would usually be identified in childhood?

*   What is the difference between a chronic condition and a degen-
    erative one?

*   What may cause fatigue for those with degenerative conditions?
```

As we are all ageing, technically we all have a degenerative condition as we cannot avoid the changes to our joints, heart, lungs etc. that come with the ageing process. In general, these are predictable and affect the majority of the population to some extent. This chapter considers the needs of those with conditions that indicate a higher level of needs, people who experience changes in their abilities, periods of remission and outcomes that significantly differ to the ageing process.

Children and young people may have a life-limiting condition, which means they are medically vulnerable and dependent on others for their care needs, but, as for some adults, their condition may not vary greatly. These would be considered chronic conditions (i.e., lasting longer than six months), and your role is to support managing changes associated with their growth.

Historically, some diagnoses, such as Duchenne muscular dystrophy or cystic fibrosis, were viewed as mainly related to childhood, but improvements in treatments and managing associated complications have increased life expectancy and longevity. Conversely, there are degenerative conditions that are rarely seen in those under the age of 18, such as multiple sclerosis, although newer diagnostic procedures mean that confirmation of a diagnosis can be made at a younger age.

When we are thinking about degenerative conditions, we include the following:

- Muscular dystrophy.

- Rett syndrome.

- Batten disease.

- Tuberous sclerosis.

- Cystic fibrosis.

- Spinal muscular atrophy.

- Multiple sclerosis.

- Motor neurone disease.

- Huntington's disease.

- Friedreich's ataxia.

But many other conditions could be added to this list. As occupational therapists don't approach assessment from the medical model, start with the person's presentation and difficulties at the point of assessment. A diagnosis is only a label, and the experience of changing abilities will differ for everyone.

Your assessment will provide you with the structure to understand the person's situation. From this you will be able to gain an understanding of their comprehension of their circumstances. Some people will have researched thoroughly and have clear objectives and an understanding of what they want to gain from your involvement. Others will prefer to focus on the here and now and are less open to discussion and planning for long-term needs.

Some parents may decide that they don't want their child to be aware of the implications of their diagnosis, and choose to limit the information that is provided to them. Restrictions limiting open discussion can make it challenging to meet a longer-term need. However, you may be able to plan for these within the scope of an adaptation through minor additions. Inclusion of a fused spur for a wash and dry toilet (or similar), for example, reduces the need for works at a later date.

The implications of a diagnosis can be overwhelming. It may be that the person or their caregivers are grieving for possibilities that are now out of reach. We all have hopes, plans and aspirations. Accepting that you or a loved one must re-evaluate these will take a period of adjustment.

There is no defined age range at which a diagnosis of a degenerative condition will be given, but this includes children and adults of working age. For children and young people, your remit will rightly focus on personal care tasks. But don't ignore other aspects of growing up, such as homework, education and family time, as well as leisure activities and interactions with peers. Don't become blinkered, and ensure you support their access to life experiences that will prepare them for adulthood.

For those of working age their identified needs will extend beyond the immediate need to manage activities of daily living. It is likely that they will have key roles and occupations that are important to them and support their involvement in family life as well as employment and leisure. The latter will usually fall outside your remit, but if you facilitate access in and out of the home, this will enable access to the community and the opportunities it affords.

Your approach must be holistic and person-centred – although you may not be working directly with a family member, you must be sensitive to their needs and signpost them to support or information services appropriately.

The implications of a diagnosis can be overwhelming. It may be that the person or their caregivers are grieving for possibilities that are now out of reach. We all have hopes, plans and aspirations. Accepting that you or a loved one must re-evaluate these will take a period of adjustment. Revisiting the 'ladder of participation' in Chapter 3, consider how you work with the person and reflect their preferred level of involvement in the adaptation process. This means that there will be times when you have to have difficult conversations, and you need to ensure that you don't raise expectations when someone is not fully accepting their situation.

Occupations and occupational performance

Once you have identified the key occupations that a person wants or needs to take part in, don't immediately think of adaptations. Can the activity be completed at a different time and/or in a different way? Would equipment be appropriate? Sometimes environmental change will be inevitable, but this can take time, so look at interim options as well.

We understand occupational performance and the impact of a barrier on the roles and routines that we need or want to do. As a person's abilities alter, they will need to adapt, both physically and mentally. Your role and recommendations are part of the wider support they will draw on. Maintaining occupations and roles is often key to a person's self-perception. They may not view themselves as disabled, which may mean they will continue to use the same methods and routines within their daily lives. Be sensitive to their preference, and respond accordingly.

Roles you may be considering and supporting include those for children. It may appear an obvious statement, but you need to support their childhood and development. The *United Nations (UN) Convention on the Rights of the Child* (UNICEF 1989) includes the right to development, family life and access to play within its principles. Development encompasses physical, emotional and educational aspects, so consider access to play for its own sake, alongside any play-based therapeutic interventions.

Family life involves all members of a household, and you should be supporting these interactions and relationships through consideration of the environment. For children there can be a challenge in that you need to support access to essential areas of the home. This may not include siblings' bedrooms or a playroom if there is access to a family room.

For adults, roles may include the parent, partner and caregiver, each of whom may need different adaptations to support the continuation of their role – and each of these is a complex combination of roles. Lim, Honey and McGrath (2022) describe a parenting role as including caregiver, nurturer, educator, protector and learner. Often these roles are completed alongside those associated with being a partner within a relationship. Roles then extend beyond nurturing and caregiving to include friend, sexual partner and shared practical roles, enabling the household to function.

Children and adults can have additional caring roles. Children and young people may care for siblings or parents, and adults may be supporting a child, their partner or other family member. In the context of this chapter, you may consider this unlikely. However, life is complex, and you may need to enable a caring role in a situation where you would expect a person to be in receipt of care rather than providing it.

Complex interactions forming family relationships and bonds are impacted by changing abilities that alter the balance of roles. Adaptations that support continuation of roles play a part in maintaining relationships and reducing stress. For those with a degenerative condition, changes may occur in a shorter timescale, and as they are not part of the ageing process, they have a greater impact on a person's emotional wellbeing.

Fatigue

Although fatigue is a symptom of some degenerative conditions, it may also result from the increased effort required to complete activities, or through altered sleep patterns due to pain or discomfort. Fatigue management can reduce the issues arising from this, and discussing how a person's day unfolds can identify where changes in routine may assist. Typically, fatigue increases as the day progresses, so managing the night-time routine will be important. If there are ground floor toilet facilities, it may be that stairs only need to be climbed in the evening, which is still a challenge if you are fatigued.

If ground floor toilet facilities are needed, this may be an opportunity to discuss long-term plans. Does the person want to remain sleeping upstairs? Is this important for them? Are they happy to start planning for an eventual move to sleep on the ground floor? For the former it may be appropriate to look to install a lift (a stairlift or through floor lift), reducing the need to use the stairs, and for the latter, consider creating a suitable bathing facility on the ground floor to meet their long-term needs.

Environmental changes to manage access to upper floors in a property can be low key, such as an additional stair rail; more complex changes include stairlifts and through floor lifts, or a significant change in sleeping arrangements, with provision on the ground floor.

Sleep is a key aspect of reducing fatigue, and an important occupation. Depending on their preference, the person may wish to continue to share a bedroom with their partner, which may impact on space for essential equipment. Alternatively, it may be that a waking caregiver is required or frequent changes of position, requiring consideration alongside equipment and transfer methods. Minimizing the disruption to a sleep pattern is part of the interaction between meeting need, supporting care provision and recognizing preference.

Bathing, toileting and personal care tasks

Bathing, toileting and personal care tasks form part of our everyday routines, and are usually private functions that we complete independently.

Children and young people who had previously developed independent personal care skills may find the need for assistance with intimate personal care tasks difficult to adjust to. Their parents and caregivers may also find this role adjustment a challenge. This may be around changing roles, recognition of a loss of ability or the management of bodily changes associated with puberty. Where a parent of a different gender has been actively involved with the child's personal care routines, they may feel that it is no longer appropriate for them to continue to do so at puberty, requiring a further adjustment in support.

Within adult relationships the need for intimate personal care may change the balance of a relationship. The person may feel uncomfortable with the role of both equal partner and caregiver. Adaptations maximizing independence or minimizing a need for assistance contribute to how people adjust and adapt.

Be responsive to the thoughts and wishes of those involved. Approach discussions with tact and discretion (a teenager may not wish to discuss their bowel movements or menstruation with a parent present or with a stranger). It may be that a caregiver is indicating that they are happy to complete these tasks, or that the person appears to accept the need for their partner's support – but is this actually the case? Are they saying this because they think it is what is expected of them? You may not be able to enable full independence, but reducing some aspects of intimate personal care may contribute to maintenance of a relationship through minimizing or delaying the need for care provision.

Offering solutions that reduce or remove the need for support for personal care can open the door to wider discussions. A person may not have considered the installation of a wash and dry toilet, or if they had, presumed that they would not be able to operate it. Advice about different types of controls, including those that can be operated remotely, may help the person regain privacy and dignity in toileting. It may be that someone is unable to operate a shower control, but rather than having someone in the room as they start showering, voice recognition options promote choice, while a remote control, which can be operated outside of the bathroom, provides privacy.

Meal preparation

What does your kitchen mean to you? It may be that it is purely a functional space where you create meals to meet your nutritional needs. Or it may hold more significance as the heart of your family home where you gather and socialize, or where you enjoy baking and cooking.

For some, skill acquisition will be the identified goal, such as for a young person with muscular dystrophy. Part of growing up is gaining independence and autonomy in everyday tasks – the ability to make a drink or a snack is encouraged by parents and caregivers. This not only provides skills but also the ability to make choices and decisions, and provides an element of control. For children and young people with a degenerative condition, the loss of control over many aspects of their lives may mean that these 'smaller' decisions have more significance than for their peers. Your response needs to be balanced and reflect their circumstances; therefore, it would not be considered reasonable and practicable to adapt an entire kitchen for someone who is not responsible for providing meals for all the family. On the other hand, ensuring that when they are at home on their own they can prepare a meal or snack is something that should be supported.

To illustrate

Parents of an eight-year-old with muscular dystrophy requested a fully adapted kitchen. He remains mobile, but is unsteady and falls frequently. Their wish was for him to have the same level of choice and ability as his siblings (who do not have the same diagnosis). He was asked what he wanted, which was to be able to prepare a drink and beans on toast.

Discussions with his parents centred round identifying a realistic solution. His parents agreed that he was not expected to do laundry or prepare full meals for the family. The solution proposed was adapting part of the kitchen, providing access and enabling preparation of snacks and drinks.

This resulted in a lowered work surface suitable for a wheelchair user, a tap with hot/cold and boiling water and a small sink. The dishwasher was moved to allow easier access, and the family installed an under-counter fridge at the end of a run of cupboards. They relocated essential items in the base units adjacent to the lowered work surface.

Maintaining access to occupations in the kitchen can offer more than fulfilling nutritional needs. Where the kitchen serves as a social hub for family meals and socialization, the focus may not be on the facilities for cooking, but on access to the room and the space within it. For those who see the kitchen as a means to an end, simply to enable access to food, maintaining occupational performance may mean provision of a lowered work surface for a microwave and kettle to prepare ready meals, snacks and drinks.

If a person considers meal preparation as a key part of their role, the loss of this occupation can have a significant impact on their self-perception, mental health and wellbeing. If meal preparation is an occupation that is integral to a person's sense of self and their role within a household, think about how to promote maintenance of this activity. Consider the role of meal preparation and mealtimes within the context of the person's culture or belief system, the options available to increase accessibility and the practicality of what needs to be achieved.

Where someone has a degenerative condition there may be a need to have challenging and difficult conversations around their changing abilities. While you can provide lowered work surfaces, adapted controls etc., a point will be reached where their symptoms, such as fatigue, tremor, grip and balance, will require them to adjust how they approach kitchen activities. It may be that ready-chopped vegetables are used or a change to the cooking method is proposed.

These conversations aren't easy or comfortable to initiate, but you have a professional responsibility to be realistic in the recommendations made. You must strike a balance between the ability of the person to accept and understand their changing abilities (now, and in the future), and a realistic and practical response to their assessed need.

Accessibility

Maintaining access in and out of a home prevents social isolation, and time spent outdoors supports mental health and wellbeing.

Take a moment to consider what you would lose if you could not leave your home. What are the occupations that are non-negotiable, or which would have the greatest impact if they were not possible?

Can we have full and enriched lives limited by our home's four walls? Many teenagers would probably say that time spent in their bedroom, connected to their peers via the internet, building communities through gaming and online activities, is sufficient. Realistically this is not a situation that should be promoted due to the risk of becoming detached from communities, the activities people enjoy or that contribute to the household.

Education and work provide opportunities to develop and become productive, as do activities such as shopping, which supports the function of a household. But it's not all work; play and leisure in all forms are key to give balance to life. Consider belief systems and culture. Gatherings serve many purposes, be that a sporting event or family gathering; they provide continued opportunities to socialize.

As independent mobility reduces, so, too, does choice and volition, with reliance on others increasing. Access options go beyond ramps and rails, although these play a part.

One note for ramps is that many people with degenerative conditions will use powered wheelchairs. Due to the torque, or simply put, the power and motion of the wheels, most temporary ramps are not suitable as they will move during use. Liaison with the wheelchair service (or discussion with the person you are supporting if they are self-funding) will mean that you can ensure that the right solution is in place at the right time.

Doors can be both enablers and barriers; if the weight of a door or the grip strength needed to operate a handle or lock means that a person cannot open the door, they are always reliant on others. As for door widths and the area needed for access through them, checking these early on in your involvement will highlight any issues that need to be addressed.

For young people there is an expectation that independent access to their community and friends will develop as they mature. If they are unable to head out to see friends, how are they able to refine their skills, ready to navigate the adult world? It may be that they have a life-limiting condition, but this should not automatically limit opportunities. An adult unable to access the community may miss out on family activities, involvement with their children's education, their own education or work opportunities, as well as being an active partner in the running of a household.

Considering how to prevent a door becoming a barrier may be low tech, such as changing a lock or handle, or extend to assistive technology, such as automatic door openers (switched or a proximity sensor, depending on the location) or digital locks. Changing the type, weight or balance of a door to meet the abilities of the person should also be considered. Doors are the entrance to our homes and personal spaces where we welcome the world into our lives. Actively deciding who you allow into your home is part of retaining control and choice. CCTV, door intercoms, smart doorbells and similar systems allow us to see who is at the door and to decide if we want to invite them in.

Fostering and maintaining independence is not limited to access and the kitchen – you will need to complete a holistic assessment and respond to the needs identified and the objectives agreed with those you are supporting.

A diagnosis of a degenerative condition may result in a high level of dependence on others, so your role is to promote the person's independence and autonomy to minimize the impact of any changes. Well-planned and timely home adaptations do more than enable functional activities, and promote the wellbeing of all household members.

14

Design and Adaptation Supporting Those with Cognitive Impairments

MARNEY WALKER

Knowledge check

* Consider a person who consistently uses the toilet during the day, but overnight frequently urinates in the airing cupboard. Why might that be?

* Consider a person who is investigated for recurrent gastric issues. Visitors to the home notice an unpleasant odour in the kitchen and usually empty the bin as they leave. What might be the connection?

(Answers to these are given at the end of the chapter.)

This chapter introduces aspects of the home environment that might impact on people living with cognitive impairments. It provides a simple explanation of cognition, cognitive impairments and who might be affected, as well as factors to consider when completing an assessment in terms of communication, and accounting for and negotiating with caregivers. Drawing on existing design principles and guidance, and aspects of the environment that might present issues, some solutions are suggested.

The primary focus is on adaptations to support people living with dementia based on evidence that simple changes support retention of abilities and influence behaviour. These solutions apply equally to people living with other cognitive impairments who experience sensory and cognitive overload. Equally, it is important to consider that each person may have other physical or sensory impairments arising from comorbidities. An emphasis is placed on *visual access*, as many of the issues and solutions impacting people with cognitive impairments apply equally to people with sight loss.

This is by no means a detailed account of all conditions causing cognitive impairments or all potential interventions, and images in this chapter illustrate key points and are not intended to be prescriptive. As an introduction to this topic we encourage you to make use of the resources at the end of the chapter, which provide sources of specialist knowledge and evidence-based guidance.

Environmental barriers

In terms of identifying environmental and attitudinal barriers to occupational performance, the Person-Environment-Occupation-Performance (PEOP) model (Baum *et al.* 2015) has particular significance. Equally, from a social model of disability perspective, both physical and social aspects affect the ability to access and use the environment. A variety of home environmental aspects act as enablers or barriers to achieving optimal occupational performance for the person, their priorities and their capabilities.

For those with cognitive impairment, the impact of environmental factors may be less easy to identify. The sensory aspects, visual and acoustic, for instance, might present a challenge. Simple changes to the way things look and feel can reduce sensory overload and support independence in everyday tasks. Creating or adapting environments that support a sense of competence and agency is the primary intention.

Cognitive impairments

At the outset, we need to understand what is meant by 'cognitive impairments'. Simply put, 'cognition' refers to processes in the brain related to how we:

- Think.
- Plan.
- Learn.
- Remember.
- Make decisions and judgements.

It also relates to how we organize and interpret *sensory information* through perception: how we see, hear, touch, taste and smell. Cognitive impairments may affect how we identify, organize and interpret sensory information. This does not necessarily mean a person with cognitive impairments cannot actively engage in most aspects of daily life. However, in a society that values intellect, negative assumptions can be made that create unnecessary attitudinal barriers to a person's self-belief.

Who might be affected: the person

There are several conditions that might impact cognition. This includes people living with dementia, mild cognitive impairment, Parkinson's disease, brain injury, substance abuse and epilepsy. In terms of neurodiversity, environmental factors considered in this chapter have relevance to people with a variety of neurological profiles who may experience what is termed *cognitive overload*, where processing information and combinations of sensory stimuli can be experienced as overwhelming and uncomfortable (BSI 2022).

Who might be affected: caregivers

For those living with cognitive impairments, the role of the primary caregiver can be significant. In conditions like dementia, where there are progressive changes, the caregiver, who is often a close family relative or friend, will be adjusting to changes in the person they have known for years. This also applies in cases of brain injury and stroke. At the time of diagnosis many refer to entering a consulting room as a spouse, sibling, son, daughter or close friend, and leaving as a caregiver.

Equality, human rights and disability rights

In the context of the Equality Act 2010, dementia is now recognized in legislation as a disability. This means that you have a duty to ensure that people living with dementia are not excluded from opportunities to participate fully in society.

When making a case for provision of adaptations, under the Care Act 2014 local authorities have a duty to promote emotional and physical wellbeing, preserve dignity and respect, ensure control over everyday life and protection from abuse or neglect, and enable participation in training, work and recreation. Guidance on how to access funding for adaptations is provided by the Equality and Human Rights Commission (EHRC) (2022) and Foundations.[1]

---

1   www.foundations.uk.com

Learning from lived experience: a person-centred approach

Each person and their situation is unique. A person-centred approach is essential to learn about the person, their home, capabilities and priorities, and which aspects of their home present an issue. This will support you to collaborate with them to find solutions that remove or minimize barriers to their independence and wellbeing.

A person-centred approach is a founding principle in occupational therapy. At the outset, where cognition is affected, invest time in ensuring you understand the person's unique situation, especially where communication may be an issue. It is essential to avoid assumptions about capabilities and capacity – the underlying principle in the Mental Capacity Act 2005 is to *assume capacity.*

Supporting a sense of identity, choice and control should be central to your approach. Capacity may vary according to each situation, and should be considered as such. Where an assessment identifies a lack of capacity, all decisions made on behalf of the person must be in their best interests. People living with cognitive impairments or experiencing cognitive overload, especially in progressive conditions, may become increasingly reliant on others for decisions about their everyday life.

It is important to be aware of the negative impacts of well-intentioned but overprotective responses. In dementia, for instance, it is recognized that negative assumptions about capabilities can accelerate the progression of the disease (Kitwood and Brooker 2019).

A strengths-based approach

While acknowledging that cognitive impairments might interfere with the ability to manage complex tasks requiring abstract thinking or time management, focusing on capabilities can maximize confidence and independence. Through an embodied knowledge and interaction with objects and materials people continue to contribute to preferred daily routines or leisure activities. An intuitive, physical, haptic and sensory response to the environment is often retained, and dexterity and coordination in familiar activities may be preserved.

Abilities vary from person to person and may fluctuate. Observation, activity analysis and simple adaptations can make it easy for the person to find and use the tools needed to complete tasks. Keeping key items in view can make a difference. This positive approach supports the ability to continue activities such as food preparation, sewing, knitting, gardening and simple DIY, and for those with early to moderate stages of dementia, continuing to drive.

Experiencing a sense of competence

Although conditions such as dementia affect cognition, this does not mean loss of identity. In acquired conditions many people retain habitual skills developed prior to a diagnosis. The development of goal-oriented cognitive rehabilitation for early-stage Alzheimer's disease (GREAT)[2] and cognitive stimulation programmes (Champagne 2018) are demonstrating people's ability to learn new skills.

Loss of ability in some aspects of life can undermine confidence in social engagement and contribute to inactivity. The right environment and opportunities enable people to be independent in many aspects of life. Paying attention to creating enabling environments supports the person to maintain and experience a sense of competence. The person may not recall what they have done earlier that day, but they can still perform quite complex skills, given the opportunity.

Embracing risk and enabling choice

The goal in occupational therapy, irrespective of condition or diagnosis, should be to enable a person to do what they want to be able to do in everyday life. This means paying attention to each person's situation, balancing risk with the benefits of continuing to participate in everyday tasks and activities. Central to this is avoiding overly restrictive practice that removes opportunities for active participation, which contributes to the person's increasing deterioration and dependence on others.

It is common for people involved in the care and support of those living with cognitive impairments to be protective, often for the very best intentions. Where a person takes much longer to complete tasks it can be easier to step in and take over. It is perhaps natural for people who have spent a lifetime together to assume that a person with dementia will need help with everything, as they adjust to changes such as difficulty with orientation or recall of recent events. The caregiver may take on responsibility for organizing household activities, financial affairs, making and tracking appointments etc., whereas, with simple adjustments, the person may be capable of managing their own personal care and a variety of household tasks.

---

2   https://sites.google.com/exeter.ac.uk/great-cr/home

Personalization

However much dementia affects the way a person's mind works, they will retain a sense of identity and a sense of their everyday likes and dislikes. This includes choosing what to wear, meal preferences, the music they enjoy and the appearance of their home. The negative impact of adaptations that appear clinical or institutional cannot be underestimated. With cognitive impairments, where a sensory response to the person's environment predominates, taking time to find out about personal likes and dislikes, including colour, can enhance a sense of agency and identity (Walker 2022).

Design principles

This chapter draws on established design principles that have been proven to support function and orientation for people living with dementia as well as other conditions impacting sensory processing: PAS 6463 (BSI 2022) and the 'Environments for Ageing and Dementia Design Assessment Tool' (EADDAT) (DSDC 2022). There is a wealth of guidance available on factors to consider and potential solutions (see 'Useful resources' at the end of this chapter). Many are more generic and derived from design of care environments or public spaces.

For occupational therapists completing home-based assessments, these principles provide a framework, but need to be adapted to domestic situations. These will assist in tailoring solutions to the person and their situation.

Key principles that are applicable to the home situation include:

- Promoting meaningful interaction and purposeful activity.

- Promoting wellbeing.

- Encouraging eating and drinking.

- Promoting mobility.

- Promoting continence and personal hygiene.

- Promoting orientation.

- Reducing unhelpful stimulation.

- Optimizing helpful stimulation.

As an occupational therapist, your approach to an assessment, irrespective of any diagnosis or condition, is person-led. Although there may be common symptoms, the experience of each person and their coping strategies will differ.

Getting to know the person

It is important to invest time in getting to know the person and allowing them to get to know you. Beware of making assumptions about capacity or capability based on your first meeting. Establishing rapport and information-gathering may take longer. The usual factors that impact on social interaction – meeting someone for the first time, social anxiety, shyness, and in an assessment, a sense of being tested – may have more of an effect on a person living with cognitive impairments and their ability to communicate. Remember that the more relaxed and comfortable we feel, the more forthcoming we are.

Introduce yourself and why you are there, and explain what you would like to know. Always include the person in the conversation, whether they have a caregiver present or not. A relaxed approach is more conducive, putting the person at ease:

- Remind the person that this is not a test.

- Face the person and make eye contact and address them by name.

- Use simple, direct, open questions.

- Allow time for a response, and listen carefully.

- It may help to mirror by repeating back what the person is saying.

- Avoid interrupting, correcting or disagreeing.

- Humour can help.

- Avoid too many questions that require factual answers, names, dates and places.

Visual communication

Objects, images and environments can be invaluable in supporting communication where word finding and narrative explanations are challenging. The advantage of a home assessment is that you can use cues from the person's familiar environment to support your questions. Where communication difficulties are significant, there are established tools that provide non-verbal ways for people to respond that may be useful, such as Talking Mats.[3]

---

3   www.talkingmats.com

Orientation and wayfinding

Simply by making it easier to see and locate key facilities, you can improve the person's orientation and function, reduce risks and their reliance on assistance, and improve their quality of life and sense of wellbeing.

A common issue for people living with dementia is *disorientation* – becoming lost, even in familiar places. An early symptom might be a person going out on an errand or a walk, and then being unable to find their way home. Innovations in location-based technologies mean that GPS tracking devices and apps can provide reassurance for a caregiver, while enabling a person to continue to have independent access to the local community. Considering this as an option must always involve ensuring that the person continues to have the capacity to consent to this, and understands risk in relation to personal and road safety.

People develop strategies (common to us all), making it easier to find their way around, for example relying on features such as a post box or a distinctive tree as landmarks. Some people wear a wrist band that prompts them to refer to a card with their caregiver's contact details or home address. This can help if they need more time when managing encounters in shops and public transport.

Recognizing home

Attention to the colour and appearance of the front door may make it stand out more clearly. Making the number larger or more visible or adding a feature near to the door can help with orientation. There is no need for these solutions to appear odd or institutional – with careful consideration for personal preferences, solutions can be inclusive and attractive. Dalke and Corso (2013) offer useful information in their book *Making an Entrance*.

Getting around the home: layout and sightlines

Even within a familiar home environment, disorientation can become an issue. Open-plan layouts with views of the kitchen, dining and lounge areas can support intuitive orientation. Leaving doors open to create sightlines serves a similar purpose. If doors are closed, the visual prompts are removed.

Being unable to find the toilet can be mistaken for incontinence. If the home layout provides clear sightlines, this can be addressed by leaving the toilet door open. A bedroom with an en suite, with a clear sightline from the head of the bed to the toilet, is ideal. Another option is sensor lighting that comes on automatically, to light the way to the bathroom.

Visuospatial perception

Cognitive impairments can influence visuospatial perception – the way we see and understand objects and spaces. People may describe the stairs as 'looking like a slide' (see Figure 10a). Attention to lighting and tonal contrast can make this easier to navigate. If it is not safe or practical to affix highlights to the nosing on the stairs (Figure 10b), you can use contrast to highlight the shape of the stairs (Figure 10c). Lighting the surface of separate treads, together with contrasting support rails, makes it easier and safer to use the stairs.

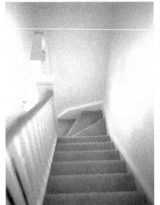
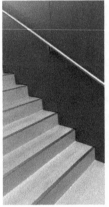
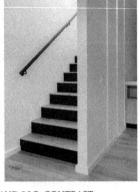

FIGURE 10A. STAIRS WITH
LITTLE VISUAL INFORMATION

FIGURES 10B AND 10C. CONTRAST
HIGHLIGHTING THE SHAPE OF THE STAIRS

FIGURES 10A–C. STAIRS: COLOUR AND DEFINITION

There may be situations when a stairlift is an identified solution. Although it is important not to adopt a blanket policy, assuming a person with a cognitive impairment lacks the capacity to use a stairlift, a risk assessment is required to establish whether the person can use or be assisted to use a stairlift. This will involve establishing whether they are able to transfer, stay on the seat while it is moving, follow instructions, and are comfortable with the experience. Giving the person and the caregiver the chance to try out a stairlift will help you all to judge whether this is a safe solution. Where the person has a progressive condition, provision of a stairlift should always include a risk assessment that factors in regular reviews. If in any doubt, seek advice; a good starting point is given in Dow (2020).

Out of sight, out of mind: making it easier to find things

Many people describe being unable to find things. Conventional storage in kitchens and bedrooms with contents concealed behind doors or drawers mean items go unnoticed. The way people cope includes leaving cupboard doors or drawers open and leaving (numerous) items out on worktops. These are strategies people naturally develop to keep things in view. If doors and drawers are closed, it may not occur to people to open them. Well-meaning caregivers may tidy away what appears to be clutter, but for the person, this means that those items have disappeared or do not exist, which may increase their anxiety.

Easy solutions include labelling drawers and cupboards with a combination of images and text. Simple drawings or photographs of key items can be effective visual prompts. Labels can be handmade, or some companies provide readymade labels. An alternative is to adapt an existing kitchen cupboard, within comfortable reach, using glazed doors and keeping key items in view (see Figure 11). Open shelving can serve the same purpose.

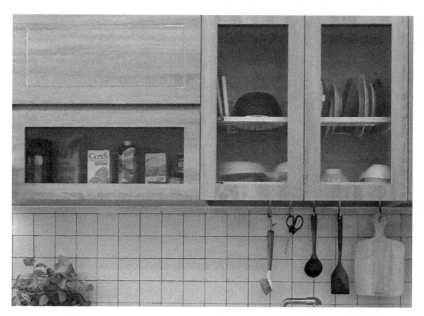

FIGURE 11. GLAZED KITCHEN UNIT

The same principle applies to containers. Frequently used items such as tea, coffee, sugar and cereal in see-through containers can provide an immediate visual cue to support independence in everyday activities (see Figure 12).

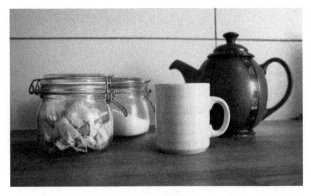

FIGURE 12. SEE-THROUGH CONTAINERS AND FAMILIAR OBJECTS
Source: Ruth Parker

Lighting

Attention to lighting can have significant benefits, with twice the normal levels of lighting recommended for those with cognitive impairments (DSDC 2013). Consider a variety of light sources that can be tailored to individual tasks and abilities, but avoid lighting that creates confusing shadows when you move into a space. Prioritise high-risk areas including steps, stairs, kitchens and bathrooms (Greasley-Adams *et al.* 2014).

Natural light

Consider maximizing existing levels of natural lighting. Curtains, blinds, window treatments and foliage can reduce light levels. Simple adjustments such as extending curtain rails so the curtains can be drawn back away from the window frame can maximize light. Views of nature, gardens and plants have significant benefits, but consider where overhanging branches might be obstructing light into the room (see Figure 13).

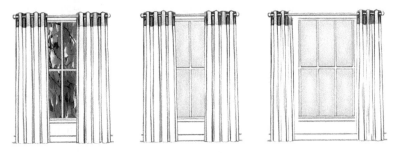

FIGURE 13. MAXIMIZING NATURAL DAYLIGHT
Source: Marney Walker

Task lighting

Pay attention to task lighting, especially in areas that might present risk, such as kitchen worktops or when shaving in the bathroom. The position and direction of lighting can support everyday activities such as food preparation and attending to personal hygiene. As many people retain skills in food preparation, making snacks or hot drinks in kitchens, consider how the worktop is lit. Lighting positioned below the wall cupboards, illuminating worktops, removes shadows, and reduces the risks of cuts and spillage that could increase the risk of falls.

Visual contrast as an enabler

It is important to understand that visual contrast does not mean using bright colours. This term refers to *tonal* and not a *colour* contrast. A visual contrast can be achieved with muted colours by using the lightness or darkness of a surface so that it shows up against the background (see Figures 14a–c). Careful attention to tonal contrast in key features of a room can act as an enabler to understanding the space and being able to find your way around.

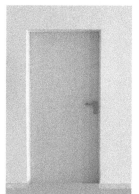 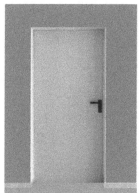 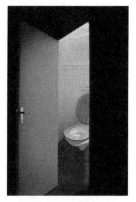

FIGURE 14A. WHITE AGAINST WHITE

FIGURE 14B. TONAL CONTRAST

FIGURE 14C. DOOR LEFT OPEN, HIGHLIGHTING ROOM USE

FIGURES 14A–C. HIGHLIGHTING DOORS
Source: Marney Walker

A light or white door will stand out against a surrounding darker wall (Figure 14b). Leaving the door open with a light on provides a visual prompt to use the toilet (Figure 14c). A toilet seat that contrasts with the white bowl can make it easier to see. Earlier research recommended red, based on age-related impairments in colour discrimination, but it is now recognized that solutions do not need to be bright colours – which may be institutional or infantile in appearance. A dark wooden toilet seat or one that coordinates with the colour scheme in a bathroom can achieve the required level of tonal contrast, and still appear homely.

In bathrooms, white sanitaryware (toilet, wash basin, bath) will merge with a white-tiled wall, whereas against a darker-tiled or painted wall they will be clearly defined and easier to locate and use (see Figures 15a and 15b).

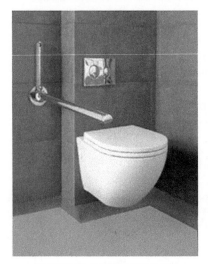 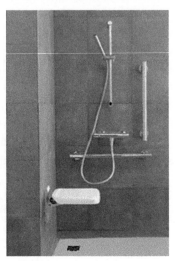

FIGURE 15A. TONAL CONTRAST
FOR THE TOILET

FIGURE 15B. TONAL CONTRAST
IN THE SHOWER AREA

FIGURES 15A–B. TONAL CONTRAST IN THE BATHROOM
Source: Kate Sheehan

Technical note: To achieve a suitable tonal contrast to make it easier to see, recognize and use key facilities, a Light Reflectance Value (LRV30) is recommended. Detailed guidance is given in PAS 6463 (BSI 2022).

Visual contrast as a barrier

- *Avoid tonal contrast on the floor:* A dark mat on a light-coloured floor will stand out, but may be perceived as a step or a hole. Transitions between rooms from a light to dark flooring will have a similar effect. Refusing to walk into a room or over a threshold can be misinterpreted as a behavioural rather than a depth perception issue.

- *Avoid strongly contrasting patterns:* Issues with depth perception can make strongly patterned 2D items appear to be 3D, and in some cases, animated. Navigating a highly patterned carpet may cause hesitancy when walking, which is sometimes misinterpreted as a physical difficulty, and increases the risk of falls (see Figures 16a and 16b).

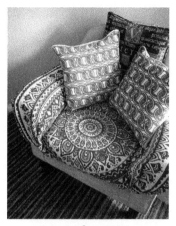

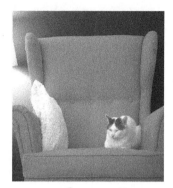

FIGURE 16A. STRONG
CONTRAST IN PATTERNS
Source: Ruth Parker

FIGURE 16B. ALTERNATIVES
WITHOUT PATTERN

FIGURES 16A–B. IMPACT OF PATTERN USE

Technical note: To avoid strong tonal contrast on flooring, a maximum of LRV5 is recommended where there are transitions between rooms or a contrast between the floor and the door mat. Detailed guidance is given in PAS 6463 (BSI 2022).

Patterns on furnishings, clothing or crockery can be confusing. People have described feeling queasy if someone is wearing a strongly striped t-shirt. A preoccupation with picking at patterns that appear to them to be floating on the surface can be a sign of issues with depth perception. Patterned crockery may appear as if there is food on the surface of a plate.

Replacing patterned clothing, furnishing and crockery with plain alternatives, while acknowledging personal preference, can resolve these issues (see Figure 17a). Creating a sense of occasion at mealtimes can support maintenance of hydration and nutrition (see Figure 17b). It is also important to consider how these solutions can be tailored to align with personal likes and dislikes, taste and style.

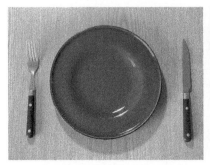

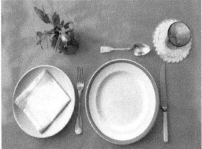

FIGURE 17A. PLAIN CROCKERY

FIGURE 17B. MAKING A
MEAL AN OCCASION

FIGURES 17A–B. PLACE SETTINGS TO PROMOTE NUTRITION
Source: Marney Walker

- *Avoid shiny surfaces:* Shiny reflective surfaces can create glare that is disturbing or disorientating. On flooring this may be perceived as a pool of water. Reflections can make the space difficult to understand (see Figure 18).

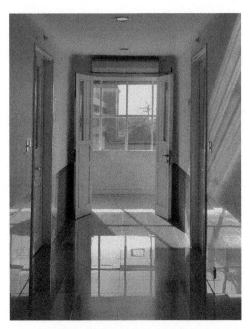

FIGURE 18. REFLECTIVE SURFACES

- *Mirrors:* Depending on the person, mirrors may become an issue. At later stages of dementia, the person may not recognize their own reflection, and believe that there is a stranger or intruder present. Removing or covering mirrors can be a solution. In shared bathrooms a small blind can be a way to conceal or reveal the mirror when needed.

Access to outdoors

Other than the benefits of regular exercise to maintain strength and mobility, there is increased evidence that daily exposure to natural daylight can reduce disturbed sleep patterns, which can be common as dementia progresses. Access to a natural environment can be part of a daily routine, providing a variety of sensory stimuli and a place for contemplation (see Figure 19). Suitable seating located in sheltered spots and features such as accessible planting and bird tables can create points of interest (Buse *et al.* 2022; Chalfont and Walker 2013).

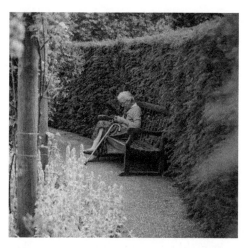

FIGURE 19. BENEFIT OF NATURAL ENVIRONMENTS

Other factors to consider:

- A view of the garden from indoors can be an invitation to go outdoors.
- How easy is it to operate the lock and the door handle?
- Does the threshold or mat present a trip hazard?
- Are support rails needed to negotiate steps or paths?
- Are surfaces of paths maintained to reduce risk of slips?

- Are there sheltered places to sit that encourage use in all weathers?

- Are there bird feeders or water features creating a point of interest?

Funding

Where there are significant cost implications, the case can be made for funding adaptations of this kind on the basis that these are recognized as environmental barriers to independent access around the home. Other than conventional routes for funding adaptations through DFGs, some local authorities have established dementia support grants in recognition of the need to fund these changes. Local authorities can use regulatory reform orders to establish ring-fenced funding for adaptations that might not fall under the usual DFG eligibility criteria but that have a significant impact on independence and wellbeing at home, such as replacement of floor coverings or safe access to the garden.

This chapter has offered a first insight into an area of practice that offers opportunities to promote continued active engagement with occupations in the home environment while minimizing the impact of cognitive impairment. Further reading and the resources below will support you in increasing your knowledge and practical solutions to help those you are supporting.

Useful resources

Alzheimer's Society (2015) *Making Your Home Dementia Friendly*: www.alzheimers.org.uk/sites/default/files/migrate/downloads/ making_your_home_dementia_friendly.pdf

Care & Repair England (2017) *Making Your Home a Better Place to Live with Dementia*: https://housingcare.org/downloads/kbase/3248.pdf

DEEP (Dementia Engagement and Empowerment Project), The UK Network of Dementia Voices: www.dementiavoices.org.uk

Department of Health and Social Care (2010) 'Nothing ventured, nothing gained: Risk guidance for people with dementia': www.gov. uk/government/publications/nothing-ventured-nothing-gained-risk-guidance-for-people-with-dementia

DLF (Disabled Living Foundation) (2019) 'Adapting your home: Managing cognitive impairment and behaviour that challenges':

https://livingmadeeasy.org.uk/dlf-factsheets/adapting-your-home-managing-cognitive-impairment-and-behaviour-that-challenges

EHRC (Equality and Human Rights Commission), 'Housing and disabled people: Your rights': https://equalityhumanrights.com/en/advice-and-guidance/housing-and-disabled-people-your-rights

EHRC (Equality and Human Rights Commission) (2018) *Your Rights to Accessible and Adaptable Housing in England*: www.equalityhumanrights.com/sites/default/files/housing-and-disabled-people-your-rights-england_0.pdf

EHRC (Equality and Human Rights Commission) (2018) *Your Rights to Accessible and Adaptable Housing in Wales*: www.equalityhumanrights.com/sites/default/files/housing-and-disabled-people-your-rights-wales.pdf

EHRC (Equality and Human Rights Commission) (2018) *Your Rights to Accessible and Adaptable Housing in Scotland:* www.equalityhumanrights.com/en/publication-download/your-rights-accessible-and-adaptable-housing-scotland

Evans, S., Waller, S., Bray, J. and Atkinson, T. (2019) 'Making homes more dementia-friendly through the use of aids and adaptations', *Healthcare 7*, 1, 43.

Garwood, S. (2017) *Are We Nearly There Yet? Enabling People with Dementia to Remain at Home: A Housing Perspective.* Dementia & Housing Working Group, Housing LIN: www.housinglin.org.uk/_assets/Resources/Housing/Support_materials/Are-We-Nearly-There-Yet.pdf

Maclean, F., Warren, A., Hunter, E. and Westcott, L. (2022) *Occupational Therapy for Dementia*. London: Jessica Kingsley Publishers.

NDA (National Disability Authority) (2015) *Dementia Friendly Dwellings for People with Dementia, their Families and Caregivers.* Centre for Excellence in Universal Design: https://universaldesign.ie/built-environment/housing/dementia-friendly-dwellings

Pearmain, H. (2018) *Embracing Risk, Enabling Choice: Guidance for Occupational Therapists*. London: Royal College of Occupational Therapists.

The King's Fund and University of Worcester (2020) 'Is your housing dementia friendly? EHE Environment Assessment Tool': https://ext-webapp-01.worc.ac.uk/kings_fund/files/ls%20your%20 housing%20dementia%20friendly.pdf

---

Having read the chapter, what do you consider to be a possible cause for the scenarios given at the beginning of the chapter?

A person who consistently uses the toilet during the day but overnight frequently urinates in the airing cupboard. Why might that be? *At night they are disorientated. All the doors are closed, making it difficult to identify which is the bathroom. This was resolved by leaving the bathroom door ajar with a light on (see Figure 14c).*

A person who is investigated for recurrent gastric issues. Visitors to the home notice an unpleasant odour in the kitchen and usually empty the bin as they leave. What might be the connection? *The fridge had been altered to an integrated unit to increase space in the kitchen. The person could not locate the fridge so they were storing fresh food in a cupboard, which was the cause of the gastric upsets. A clear label on the fridge and prompts from visitors made identification of the fridge easier.*

15

Adaptations to Reduce the Impact of Frailty

Knowledge check

* What do you consider 'frailty' to be? Do you have an image of a little 92-year-old with a walking frame in mind? What is it that constitutes frailty?

* Which of the following are the identifiers proposed by Fried *et al.* (2001):

    (a) Aged 80+ years?

    (b) Weakness?

    (c) Slow walking speed?

    (d) Frequent falls?

    (e) Low physical activity?

    (f) Self-reported exhaustion?

    (g) Impaired cognitive abilities?

    (h) Incontinence?

    (i) Unintentional weight loss?

(The answer is provided at the end of the chapter.)

Professor John Young (2013) defines frailty in medicine as referring to those older people who are at higher risk of adverse outcomes, which includes disability, falls, conditions resulting in admission to hospital, or which may result in a need for long-term care. As with all conditions, frailty can be viewed as a spectrum, with individuals with mild frailty presenting very differently from those with severe symptoms. Revisiting that image of a 92-year-old, if they remain active and generally well, with no comorbidities, then even with their advanced age they would be considered as having mild frailty. This could be compared with someone 20 years younger who has osteoarthritis, chronic obstructive airways disease and diabetes, who we would consider as having severe frailty.

> It is worth mentioning that the impact of the ageing process and disease will vary between individuals, so a referral that lists numerous conditions may not be for someone who presents with severe frailty.

The ageing process affects the whole body – eyesight and hearing become less acute, there is reduced ability to retain information, and orthopaedic changes reduce range of movement and cause discomfort or pain. In addition to this, when someone becomes frail, they are likely to become less active, resulting in deconditioning, which places them at higher risk of falls or injury. Each of these changes may be minor but in combination may cause dependency on others to manage activities of daily living, leading to reduced involvement in occupations and limiting activities outside of the home. This means that this population is more likely to be known to both health and social care – typically across several departments or services that, in an ideal world, will coordinate responses to identified needs.

Tools are available to assess for frailty, providing a consistent approach and shared language. Dolenc and Rotar-Pavlič (2019), for example, offer a selection.

Fatigue and energy levels

With reduced energy and increased discomfort, some people reduce their level of physical activity, choosing to spend increased time sitting in an armchair. Sedentary behaviour can seem a sensible response to fatigue, but is not recommended. Responding to this by promoting access to essential facilities, perhaps the use of only one or two rooms on the ground floor of a property, appears to be a pragmatic option. But actually, no, the impact of reduced physical activity is further muscle loss affecting the whole body, including cardiac muscles, as well as increasing the likelihood of osteoporosis. Therefore, your role is to support the maintenance of physical activity, finding a balance between 'enough' movement and preventing over-exertion. An example of this is the need to climb stairs. If you remove the need to climb stairs by ground floor living, the installation of a stairlift or through floor lift, these options reduce the associated health benefits. Climbing stairs strengthens more than just the leg muscles; it also gives the heart and lungs a workout. The effort required burns calories, which assists with weight management. Utilizing activity or task analysis you can determine that there are additional benefits as the process of climbing stairs requires balance and coordination (bilateral movement patterns), plus agility, strength and concentration. Therefore, removing the need to climb stairs can have a negative impact on the person's health and wellbeing.

This is not to say that you should promote this for all. Your holistic assessment and understanding of positive risk-taking will enable you to assess if this is an activity that should be supported, such as by providing an additional stair rail or enhanced lighting. Supporting continued activity, albeit often at a reduced pace, can be enabled by additional rails, half-steps and similar small changes. As part of your approach, look at equipment and furnishings, check that the height of seating and beds is optimal, and identify if equipment such as raisers or toilet frames are required. This sits alongside advice on energy management and pacing through liaison with health colleagues such as physiotherapists and GPs.

A thought: is a trolley a facilitator or a barrier to promotion of activity? It may be that it is utilized as intended, ensuring the safe transfer of items between the kitchen and sitting room. But how often do we see trolleys next to a chair laden with everything that might be needed? Yes, that is very convenient, but think of all those lost opportunities to go and get a pen, tissue, notepad, book...

Falls

A key area of support for those with frailty is falls prevention. The Office for Health Improvement and Disparities (2022) provides statistics that highlight the impact of falls on individuals and on the services supporting them after a fall: fragility fractures are estimated to cost these services £4.4 billion – a staggering amount that is dwarfed by the personal impact on those who are injured. They advise that 'Falls and fractures in older people are often preventable' (Office for Health Improvement and Disparities 2022), which is where occupational therapists play a role.

First and foremost, consider the person. As you visit them in their home, is there anything that gives you concern as you observe them moving between rooms? Has their presentation changed since your last visit? Do they have a visual impairment? Do they have a diagnosis such as Parkinson's disease, or are they on multiple medications (polypharmacy)? It may be that you observe something that you feel needs addressing. You may offer them advice, signpost them to a service or refer them for assessment such as by a physiotherapist (subject to local referral processes, of course).

Once you have noted your observations of the person, consider their home environment. Look at hazards that contribute to slips, trips and falls, such as lighting, rugs and pets. Some slight changes can have an immediate impact, such as increasing light levels and removing rugs. Although pets are not something that can be removed, advising owners that they or their toys can be a trip hazard goes a little way to mitigating the associated risks.

Understanding a person's day and night-time routines will help with identifying where changes can be made. There may be a large step at the back door, but if they never go out into the garden, installing grab rails and a half-step will not reduce the chance of a fall. There are activities that increase the risk of a fall, such as using the stairs or transfers during bathing. Additional stair rails increase safety on the stairs, and safe bathing can be promoted through changes such as the installation of grab rails or a level-access shower, depending on the level of assessed need and discussion with the person.

Nutrition and hydration

Food is fuel and essential to good health, as is remaining hydrated. The British Nutrition Foundation (2022) advises that as we age, we are more vulnerable to dehydration. Causes include a decreased sensation of thirst, loss of cognitive ability (recall), orientation in time, swallowing difficulties and the need for assistance and medications, especially diuretics. The outcome of being dehydrated can include increased risk of pressure areas, reduced renal function, dizziness and fatigue.

Food provides the nutrients we need for good health. The ageing process can affect our sense of taste, reducing our enjoyment of meals, and from this the inclination to spend time preparing dishes. Those who use less energy burn fewer calories and this, in turn, reduces the need for food. Adapting an approach from which meals move from freshly prepared and varied dishes to ready-meals can adversely affect nutrition, so you have a part to play in the promotion of independence in this occupation.

The first step is to enable access to and from the kitchen; this is part of your wider consideration, but with the addition of how food and drink is carried safely through to where it is to be consumed. Once in the kitchen area mobility and access to different areas need to be considered, but you also need to respond to a person's stamina or fatigue level. Is there space to sit to rest or during food preparation? Or would it be better to prepare food in another area, where there is space to sit? Adaptations to consider are lowered areas of work surfaces or height-adjustable ones to enable varied work positions, which also supports use by other family members.

Grip strength may be reduced, making manipulation of handles, taps or controls difficult. Changing these may resolve the issue, but if shoulder range of movement is restricted, then considering the position of taps and their design is indicated. Sensor taps require no grip and can be operated at a distance; lever taps with paddle handles are easier to operate than taps with rotating heads, but recommending longer length levers might be required. The ability to lift or relocate saucepans, a kettle or heavy dishes may be impacted by both grip and muscle weakness. The use of small items of equipment, such as mesh baskets within saucepans or kettle tippers, reduces effort. Ensuring that there are work surfaces either side of the hob or adjacent to the oven that are suitable for hot pans to be moved on to removes some of the risks and difficulties linked with pan weight and hot food or liquids. It may be appropriate to alter the design of a hob to one with a low profile, so there is less height difference between the two areas.

Although changes can be viewed as beneficial, if there is a loss of cognitive ability associated with frailty, then the changes, while practical, may further reduce kitchen activity, as their use may not be intuitive for a person. The change from knob controls to a sleek flat surface with touch-responsive controls may mean that the hob is no longer used.

If cognition is affected, then reminders or alarms can be used to promote or maintain routines around nutrition and hydration. Smart speakers can be programmed to provide reminders to eat and drink. To reduce disorientation, reminders can be recorded by those familiar to the person.

Smoke or heat detectors are recommended within any kitchen. A fire safety check is usually part of the offer by local Fire and Rescue Services, which often have schemes that install these without charge.

Incontinence

Veronese *et al.* (2018) advise that urinary incontinence is twice as common in older people with frailty than with their peer group. Causes include:

- The ageing process, with pelvic floor and bladder muscles becoming weaker, including prolapse of pelvic organs.

- Neurological changes increasing muscle activity or bladder sensitivity, including those associated with medical conditions such as Parkinson's disease, diabetes and multiple sclerosis.

- Changes linked to the prostate gland.

- Medications with a diuretic effect.

- Functional difficulties, which mean that a person cannot reach the bathroom in time.

Incontinence may affect the skin condition of the lower body, increasing the chance of infection. Reduced fluid intake may lead to dehydration, causing an increase in concentration of urine, which irritates the bladder lining, causing or increasing incontinence. Dehydration increases the risk of a urinary tract infection (UTI), which also causes incontinence but can also present with other symptoms including confusion. This, in turn, may reduce fluid intake, a cycle that will result in multiple issues.

Physical inability to access a toilet facility may cause incontinence when there is no direct bladder or bowel issue. A commode is a solution that may partially resolve the problem, but the waste will need to be disposed of. If a person is unable to mobilize to reach the toilet, then you can assume they are likely to have difficulty removing a commode pan and disposing of the waste.

It is highly likely you will be able to identify a problem with incontinence through your sense of smell, identifying a stale urine smell from clothing, furnishing or flooring. However, the smell could result from incontinence products the person has been unable to move to the external rubbish. Alternatively, a strong urine smell could be due to an untreated UTI. It may be a difficult conversation to initiate, but one you must have, as your response will vary depending on the cause of the incontinence.

Temperature regulation

Temperature regulation is essential to the maintenance of health. As we age, our ability to recognize our body temperature is reduced. While we usually think about the impact of low temperature and hypothermia, we also need to consider excessive heat.

First, though, low temperatures: hypothermia is a body temperature below 35°C; symptoms include pale or dry skin, slow breathing, confusion and tiredness, all of which could be disregarded as an inevitable part of ageing and frailty. An experiment reported by BBC Radio 4's *Inside Health* (Gallagher 2022) highlighted that at an ambient temperature of 18°C our body starts to work to protect our core temperature. This is achieved through changes including vasoconstriction, which directs blood away from our extremities, an effect more marked in females than males. Readings taken at a room temperature of 10°C after just 30 minutes demonstrated:

- A reduction of 20% of blood flow to the brain.

- Raised mean arterial blood pressure.

- Increased breathing rate.

- Higher carbohydrate burn level.

- Temperatures in the extremities lower by 2°C.

- Increased time taken to complete a cognition puzzle.

This demonstrates that although the person's core temperature remained at 37°C and they were not hypothermic, there was, nonetheless, a significant impact.

Higher energy costs during the colder months, and income restricted to a pension or benefits, means that many people are unable to heat their homes adequately. Additionally, if they have lived in their home for a lengthy period and are used to the heating system, they may not consider (or be able to afford) that it needs to be upgraded. How does this relate to adaptations? Your first option may be signposting. This could be to grants to replace the heating system or support that energy suppliers have in place for vulnerable customers. Assess the person's ability to operate the controls – boiler, radiator or gas or electric fires – and adapt these to a more suitable design. There are still properties with back boilers or systems run from wood burning stoves or with storage heaters. For these the issue may not be the ability of the person to operate them, but more that there will be variations of temperature throughout a 24-hour period.

The general condition of a property contributes to thermoregulation. If windows and doors are in need of repair or replacement, signpost to available support or include this within a **recommendation for adaptation** within your case notes. It may be that only rooms that are used regularly can be upgraded, but this will assist with maintaining warmth, especially in the sitting room and bedroom, where people tend to be least active.

> A note of caution: If a person relocates their bedroom to a ground floor room heated by a ventless gas fire, the fire must be decommissioned due to risks associated with carbon monoxide (HSE 2022). Many landlords will insist that a gas fire is decommissioned regardless of type, to remove any risk.

Overheating (hyperthermia) is just as relevant as hypothermia, but is a concern throughout the year. The impact of climate change has meant that recent summers have been noticeably hotter – in July 2022 England recorded a 40°C temperature for the first time since records began (Met Office 2022). During cooler months, overheating may result from a person's inability to recognize that they are in an adequately heated room. If the room temperature is too high, the symptoms that a person may exhibit include cold or clammy skin, tiredness or exhaustion, weakness or dizziness, although these symptoms can be attributed to other causes. In this instance a smart speaker can highlight when an optimum temperature is reached, and offer prompts to open windows to ventilate the room.

An additional consideration is the risk of burns if the heating is set too high or supplemented by freestanding heat sources such as oil-filled portable radiators or fan heaters. Direct contact with heat may not be recognized due to reduced skin sensitivity, as may the effect of hot air from fan heaters, either causing burns or increasing the fragility of skin, which has already been affected by the ageing process.

A scenario to consider

A 90+year-old couple: she remains active, with minimal health conditions; he is frail, with comorbidities including asthma, osteoarthritis, impaired cognition and visual impairment. He wants the central heating fully on, with windows and doors closed. His wife finds the house stifling, but if windows or doors are opened, he becomes agitated. He will not put on additional layers to compensate. He reports that he is always exhausted and has dizzy episodes, which his wife attributes to the heat.

Social isolation

With a reduction in mobility, anxiety about falls or cognitive changes, there is an increased risk of social isolation. You can support people through sign-posting to appropriate services, but consider the barriers that their home may present. A person's reluctance to leave their home could be linked to their difficulty in maintaining personal hygiene. If they feel that they are unable to wash or bathe effectively, they may feel that they have an unpleasant body odour, even if this is not the case. Supporting their access to bathing and toileting may remove this perceived barrier.

If support to engage in activities in the community is available, access to and from the home needs to enable this. It isn't appropriate to provide a dropped kerb and off-road parking for rare trips by car, but ensuring there are grab rails, steps of an appropriate height or a ramp for wheelchair users will remove some physical barriers, and hopefully promote increased time spent in the community.

Caregiver support

Frailty increases the need for support from others. This may be from an informal caregiver, generally a family member, or formal caregivers, who are contracted for set hours and activities. Your role is to consider how the environment can be altered to enable this care. Bathrooms are often the smallest room in the house, and if this does not enable the caregiver to give the support needed, there is a risk of injury to both the person receiving support and the caregiver. Adaptations will then need to reflect the need for a second person in a space usually occupied by an individual, and the need for equipment such as commodes, changing or shower stretchers, toilet frames etc.

Prevention of hospital admission and long-term care

While adaptations will rarely have a direct impact on admission to hospital due to a change in a person's health, they do have a part to play in support-ing the maintenance of health and wellbeing, both physical and mental, and minimizing the risk of injury. These indirectly reduce the likelihood of admission to hospital and also the need to move to long-term residential or nursing care.

The ageing process cannot be predicted, and the presence of comorbidities can combine, resulting in frailty. The home environment may present barriers that exacerbate a person's difficulties; your skills and knowledge will enable you to address these barriers. If a referral and assessment present a list of diagnoses and a home environment with numerous barriers, you could focus on the negatives. Adopting a strengths-based approach, where you build on positives, working alongside adaptations and sources of support, means you promote choice and involvement in the adaptation process. Remember that impaired cognition does not remove capacity or prevent decision-making. Promotion of positive outcomes, maintenance of routines and independence and the ability to live a full life should be the aspiration and expectation of all those working with this population, with adaptations contributing to the wider support systems available.

Answer to the knowledge check

For those who didn't resort to the internet for the knowledge check, the answers are: (b), (c), (e), (f) and (i). This is one approach and perhaps over-simplistic, used here to pose a question rather than identify a preferred approach.

16

Supporting People with Different Body Shapes

Knowledge check

* How many descriptors are there for different body shapes of obese people?

* What physical impact might a person of excessive height have when picking an item up from a low level?

* What is the maximum safe working load that can be achieved via a tracked hoist?

* How could you reduce the impact of restricted upper limb length in the kitchen?

Body shape

People come in different shapes and sizes, and design of housing adaptations must consider this. Altered diets and access to healthcare have resulted in the average height of adults increasing significantly, with a height of 6'6" not being considered unusually tall. Growth rates vary, and a person's height may reflect their parents' stature or genetics. Some people may have a short stature, defined as 'having a final adult height of 4'10" or less due to a medical condition' (RGA 2022). The Restricted Growth Association (RGA) advises that those with restricted growth have a variety of body shapes that are either proportionate or disproportionate to height. There are also some medical conditions that result in significant growth rates – at the time of writing (2022) the *Guinness Book of Records* advised that the tallest living person is currently 8'2" (Atwal 2022).

This doesn't tell the whole story. A person's height is influenced by a range of factors, some naturally occurring or resulting from medical or surgical interventions, including side effects from medications provided in childhood or due to amputation of lower limbs.

Not only are people growing in height, but we are also seeing a marked change in body shape and in obesity rates. (We use the term 'obese' here rather than 'bariatric', which relates to the treatment of obesity, or 'plus size', which is a descriptor of clothes size.) With weight gain, there may be changes in body size, and shape will vary beyond the traditional descriptors such as 'apple' or 'pear'.

Body shapes of obese people can be:

- *Proportional:* With even weight gain.

- *Bulbous gluteal:* Weight gain is focused around the buttocks, resulting in a posterior-protruding shape.

- *Pear:* Weight is distributed unevenly, concentrated in the lower body area.

- *Apple:* Weight gain is situated around the centre of the body.

- *Apple ascites:* Accumulated fluid, causing an extended, rigid abdomen.

- *Apple panniculus:* A hanging mass of subcutaneous fat in the lower abdomen, often referred to as an 'apron'.

- *Pear abduction:* Excess tissue on the inner thighs, resulting in hip and thigh abduction that alters gait as well as body shape.

- *Pear adduction:* Excess tissue on the outer thighs, which creates a significant hip width.

- *Anasarca*: Generalized increase in body size due to excess fluid.

These are changes to body shape, but oedema or lymphoedema can affect a single limb or part of a limb, and uni- or bilateral changes to limb shape need to be taken into consideration when designing spaces.

This returns us to the person-centred approach where the person's circumstances are considered and responded to. Your assessment and professional reasoning will assist you in enabling occupations of purpose and choice. Considerations include reach, flexibility and symptoms associated with body shape. A person with excessive height may experience postural hypotension when reaching for something at floor level, and someone with shorter limb length may find the depth of a kitchen work surface a challenge.

Where reach is identified as a barrier, assistive technology can facilitate opening windows, for example, especially in the kitchen and bathroom where they are often located above the sink or bath. Wall cupboards can be fitted with pull-down shelves or mounted on tracks so they can be lowered, or the kitchen could be fitted with base units only.

For those of short stature the position of light switches can be a barrier, especially for young children. You should be led by the person's preference, and also the needs of others in the household. The person may prefer to have steps or stools located to enable reach, or there may be family household members with significant differences in height. Assistive technology can compensate, or sometimes a simple change can resolve an issue, such as increasing the length of a bathroom light pull cord.

Changes in body shape can also result from scoliosis and kyphosis. These, in turn, as with other conditions affecting body shape, may result in comorbidities including impaired lung function, digestive issues or heart conditions, which must be taken into consideration.

Resolving issues relating to body shape requires lateral thinking, but the room-specific chapters in this book (Chapters 20 to 23) provide examples of adaptations so you are not starting from scratch.

This chapter continues with a focus on supporting access and equipment for the obese person, which reflects the specific knowledge needed to safely complete adaptations that take into account safe working loads and structural changes that are not required for those whose weight is within the typical range.

Access issues

If home access becomes a challenge, then a person may become less inclined to socialize outside of the home, or their world contracts to partial use of the space. Lack of socialization affects mental health, and reduced physical activity affects all areas of physical health. Additionally, if someone has difficulty in leaving their home, they may no longer be able to attend medical appointments, further impacting on their health and wellbeing.

If a person's body shape and weight is such that they can no longer fit through the doors, an emergency reaction to a medical crisis requires drastic measures. Removing windows or demolishing part of a wall may be a practical solution, but it does not afford privacy or dignity. A proactive multi-agency approach can minimize the need for such responses, and you can contribute to this through consideration of emergency egress when supporting an obese person.

If a person has difficulty passing through their home's main exit, then it stands to reason that the access points to the main rooms in the house should be reviewed. Widening doors can be achieved through a wider door set or fitting one-and-a-half or double doors, but it is not just doors that need to be considered. Space between kitchen units and hallways can be limited, reducing access. Removing one run of kitchen units will reduce storage but increase access. If a hallway is too narrow, relocating a radiator or altering doors so they open into adjoining rooms rather than the hallway may provide sufficient space. Open-plan living may be a solution if it is not possible to create sufficient space. Where routes between rooms are suitable you may need to identify appropriate resting places to manage breathlessness or fatigue. Where a hallway is a significant length, it can be a challenge to identify how to provide a rest point without reducing the available width.

Property construction

Domestic properties are constructed for those of a typical weight, and so advice may be required on strengthening stairs, walls, floors and ceilings. Stairs are usually constructed of wood, and may be neither wide nor robust enough for use. Cumulative weight, such as the person and their specialist bed, or when in the bath, may require floors to be strengthened regardless of which floor they are on. Joists are obscured from view, but the type used in construction will impact on adaptation options including the installation of tracked hoists. Walls may need steel plates added to enable the installation of grab rails. Flats and apartments may pose additional challenges due to their construction and number of shared walls, floors and ceilings. This is not to say that a mid-terrace or single-storey property will not present challenges – just different ones. Luckily for you, you only need an awareness of potential issues, as the surveyor or structural engineer will advise on the appropriate structural changes needed.

Weight limits relate not only to the fabric of the building; ramps and rails also have recommended maximum user weights. If specifying a design or type, you will be responsible for ensuring your recommendation is appropriate. An alternative approach is to advise 'installation of x with a maximum user weight of y'. And don't forget that ramps will need to consider the person, any mobility equipment plus any caregiver supporting them – which is cumulatively quite a considerable weight. Floor fixed rails or drop-down rails with a supporting leg may provide more suitable options for support than wall-mounted grab rails, but installation methods will reflect the property's construction.

Space

Space is often a challenge for those with disabilities, and for the obese person you need to consider their size, mobility, space for equipment, plus space for caregivers. The number of caregivers needed to enable care provision will increase where a person's ability to reposition themselves is reduced and where limbs are significantly heavier.

Tracked hoists can be installed with maximum user weight limits of 50 stone. Installed in tandem, this can increase to 72 stone as long as the building's construction is suitable. Tracked hoists require a smaller space for manoeuvring, and a powered traverse will reduce the load a caregiver will need to handle during transfers.

Where wheeled equipment is used for support or transfers, a larger turning circle will be needed – not just because the equipment is larger, but also because of the effort required to initiate and maintain momentum. This is affected by the floor surface, where carpet will create greater resistance than a wood or laminate finish.

Room sizes are usually dictated by the design of a property, but Housing LIN offers some advice on this area of provision.[1]

Toileting and bathing

Thinking about specific activities, access to toileting and bathing provides us with the most frequent requests for adaptation.

Toileting advice includes:

- The distance of the toilet from adjacent walls should take into consideration the body shape of the person.

- Providing a minimum distance of 600mm between the centre line of the toilet bowl and the wall allows for caregiver access (but consider the point above).

- Wall-hung toilets are not appropriate due to maximum user weight and their low tolerance for those who are unable to lower themselves to sitting in a controlled manner.

---

1   See www.housinglin.org.uk/Discuss/download/1599

- Higher toilet seat heights aid rising to stand.

- Basins, towel rails and radiators should be positioned away from the toilet, reducing the risks associated with their use as a transfer aid.

- There are toilets and toilet seats with higher user weights on the market. Designs such as the Big John toilet seat may offer more comfort during toileting.

- Cleansing after toileting may be impeded by body shape, so a wash and dry toilet may be appropriate, subject to maximum user weight.

When assessing for bathing options, consider:

- The cumulative weight of the person, equipment and water when using a bath.

- The pressure directed down through the feet or base of equipment in use and the strength of the base it is placed on (think acrylic baths or shower trays).

- The ability of the person to dry themselves after bathing. A wall or ceiling-mounted body dryer may be appropriate.

- Longer shower hoses allow for reduced range of movement and wider girth.

- Basins should be mounted on a pedestal or robust unit.

- Showering may be a more practical solution considering the above, the person's transfer ability, caregiver support and the ability to ensure all areas of the body are cleansed.

- Increased perspiration can cause skin folds to become inflamed and infected, highlighting the need for accessible bathing facilities.

Temperature regulation

Obesity affects regulation of body temperature, the impact of this being increased perspiration and susceptibility to heat stress. There is a risk of dehydration if the person cannot access regular hydration or restricts their fluid intake as access to a toilet is difficult. Heat stroke or heat exhaustion may result from the body's reduced ability to maintain an appropriate core temperature, exacerbated in recent years by the increase in frequency of heatwaves in the UK. Reduced mobility or range of movement may mean that a person is unable to open windows or doors to regulate room temperature. Assistive technology or automation linked to thermostats can be considered. Alternatively, air conditioning units may be required in frequently used rooms.

Floor finishes

Floor surface was referenced above, in relation to the use of wheeled transfer and mobility equipment. The choice of floor finish needs to consider durability and resistance, but also the effect of the downward force of static items of furniture and equipment. This may result in deep indentations or breaks in the continuity of the surface. At best this is a trip hazard if the furniture or equipment is relocated, but if the downward pressure breaks the seal created by the slip-resistant surface used within a level-access shower, for example, then the implications are far greater. A leak will impact the integrity of the floor, the ceiling of the room below and retain moisture within the shower room, increasing the chance that it will become mouldy and musty.

Body shapes and types differ widely, and your role is to consider these alongside all the other aspects of a person's assessed needs. Body shape in itself is not a disability, but it can be disabling, and so forms part of a holistic assessment. This chapter has, in the main, focused on the obese person, but any body shape that falls outside the 'norm' will face barriers as our environments are designed to meet the needs of the many. While the evidence base supporting practice is limited, often focusing on hospital or residential locations, useful learning points can be applied within domestic dwellings. Occupational therapists are key to ensuring that the barriers from this design approach are removed, facilitating independence, choice and occupations for those where the design of the built environment does not consider their diverse body shape or build.

Useful resources
de Lange, L., Coyle, E., Todd, H. and Williams, C. (2018) 'Evidence-based practice guidelines for prescribing home modifications for clients with bariatric care needs.' *Australian Occupational Therapy Journal* 65, 2, 107–114: https://pubmed.ncbi.nlm.nih.gov/29314054

Health and Safety Executive (2007) 'Risk assessment and process planning for bariatric patient handling pathways': www.hse.gov.uk/research/rrpdf/rr573.pdf

Kent County Council (2014) 'Extra care design principles': www.kent.gov.uk/__data/assets/pdf_file/0017/14255/Final-Extracare-Design-Principles.pdf

Peninsula Health Care Network (2015) 'Occupational therapy evidence-based practice guidelines for the prescription of bariatric home modifications': www.homemods.info/Download.ashx?File=eb7587f2804351b2c4bb3647e92376b&C=31342c3333342c30

17

Adapting for Safety

Minimizing the Impact of Behaviours that Challenge

AMMELIA MAY AND RUTH PARKER

Knowledge check

* What is meant by 'stimming'?

* What is a Dutch door (stable door)?

* Fire escape windows may not have locks fitted. True or false?

* Name a condition where a person may choose to eat non-food items.

* Why do we adapt to manage behaviours that challenge – is it for the individual or for those who care for them?

* At what age does the Mental Capacity Act 2005 apply?

* Name two ways an adaptation can support de-escalation.

Before we begin, restrictive practice will be a theme throughout this chapter. It is something that will need to be considered, as there is a need to balance the safety of the individual with the safety of others. However, we also have a responsibility to promote choice and freedom of action. Chapter 6 on legislation provides a background to some of the considerations you will have to take into account when adapting environments in response to behaviours that challenge.

What is a behaviour that challenges?

There is no list to confirm if the behaviour identified as an issue meets this definition of a 'behaviour that challenges'. Nor is there a level for each behaviour that says it becomes one that challenges. Some will reflect societal norms, some the risk of injury, and others the ability of those around an individual to accept (or ignore) a behaviour. Behaviours that cause injury to a person, damage property or the environment clearly challenge when an action is directed towards a person, but also affect those observing the behaviour.

Where behaviours are judged against societal norms, be aware that these are not static – some individuals may find it difficult to accept that a behaviour does not need to be prevented or modified. Therefore, it can be said that some behaviours that challenge are more an issue for those observing them than for the individual exhibiting the behaviour.

Causes of challenging behaviours include frustration or an inability to communicate a need rather than an intention to cause harm or damage. There are behaviours that provide a preferred sensation for an individual, including spinning, flapping, rocking and banging, which are often referred to as 'stimming'. These may not result in injury or destruction of property, but the impact on others may mean that they are described as challenging. A feature of these behaviours is that the individual presenting the behaviour does not often appreciate the risks associated with their actions, and has a lack of awareness of the impact on others.

Do not presume that a behaviour that challenges will always be present, or that it will increase in frequency or severity. With maturity, through therapeutic support and the identification of sensory preferences, behaviours can be minimized or effectively managed.

The impact of behaviours extends beyond the immediate outcome of the behaviour itself. Beyond the behaviour consider the risk of injury and possible destruction of property. As people generally don't live alone, behaviours that challenge also affect all those in the household. This could be through high levels of stress, fear of injury or aggression or lack of sleep. These behaviours affect life outside of the house, impacting education, employment and leisure opportunities. The risk of social isolation is high, as those within a support network may feel unable to manage behaviours, reducing the help available and opportunities. Issues may arise with neighbours if a behaviour is not managed effectively, and can escalate to involvement of the police, safeguarding or housing officers.

Examples where neighbours may be affected by challenging behaviour include:

- *Banging:* Noise levels – when there is repetitive banging on a radiator, for example.

- *Water:* A fascination with water may be a flood risk, especially when living in a flat.

- *Clothing:* Windows and gardens mean neighbours may be exposed to nudity if clothing isn't tolerated.

What outcome are you working towards?

When considering solutions, you are aiming to meet the needs of the individual who has been referred. However, this is in addition to balancing support for those around them and safety for all. The aim is to minimize the impact of behaviours that challenge and to reduce risk, but also to acknowledge that removing access to one thing may redirect the behaviour towards something else. For example, padding a bedroom wall removes feedback from contact with a wall. This may direct this behaviour to another location in the home (but it wouldn't be practical to pad the whole property).

Environmental adaptations may not change the behaviour itself, but reducing frequency or impact strengthens the resilience of those around the person, such as by enabling parents or caregivers to have more restful sleep, or reducing their stress and anxiety. Therefore, prior to planning adaptations, consider all other options to reduce the behaviour itself. This enables more positive outcomes for the wellbeing of the person, increases household members' resilience and reduces stress. Early intervention to minimize the behaviour itself, or the impact of the behaviour, reduces the likelihood of social isolation, as the person is no longer limited to their immediate adapted environment.

However, accessing support for sensory-processing difficulties or behaviours that challenge is varied and often limited. Advice and support is available from websites and social media, which can supplement local services that may offer face-to-face or telephone support or signposting to other sources of support. Independent therapists work in this area of practice; however, their services attract a cost, and may be unaffordable for some families.

Parents and families should be encouraged to try strategies for a period of time, and may find it helpful to keep a diary or log to provide evidence.

This can then be used as part of a risk evaluation to determine the likelihood of a challenging behaviour and associated level of risk.

Behaviours that challenge often result from an inability to communicate thoughts, feelings and preferences. Before changing the environment it is worth considering how communication can be promoted. This could be through a variety of methods (e.g., a paper-based scan-and-select system, technology such as eye-gaze, or vocalizations and facial expressions). A starting point is to ask how communication is managed at settings outside of the home. As communication includes preparation for an activity, especially if it falls outside of a routine, taking time to prepare the person beforehand may prevent or reduce behaviours. There may not be a suitable option, but it should be considered when completing adaptations that are outside of a person's normal routine. One approach used to prepare a teenager with autism and Duchenne muscular dystrophy for the planned adaptation was to create a LEGO® model of what his new bedroom would look like.

Another factor causing behaviours that challenge is sensory-processing difficulties, through either an under- or oversensitivity to the seven senses: visual, auditory, gulfactory (taste), touch, proprioception, vestibular and interoception. A person may either be sensory-seeking or sensory-avoiding, and display this as behaviours that challenge to balance their sensory processing to an optimal state. It is often difficult to determine what sense the person is having difficulty with at any moment, particularly if they have non-verbal methods of communication. Complicating matters, a person can be both under- and oversensitive in different areas and at different times of the day.

Families and caregivers may know that a person has a high pain threshold or likes messy play, for example, but may not be aware of all seven senses or that they have specific sensory-processing difficulties, potentially causing the behaviours that challenge. Sensory-processing difficulties present challenges in both the impact of exhibited behaviours and identification of solutions to minimize the associated risks, and to this we add the impact on the person while adaptations are being completed.

Assessing behaviours outside the home

While it is useful to evaluate behaviours in different environments, it is also important to remember that stimuli around them will differ. Teachers and day centre staff are likely to have more resilience as they work set hours. People can sometimes self-regulate to some degree when away from the home, reducing the frequency of a behaviour. However, their 'sensory cup' is filled throughout the day and may then 'overspill' when they return home.

Picking your battles...

Families, in partnership with professionals, may need to consider which behaviours are acceptable overall and which require addressing. It can be difficult for people close to the person exhibiting a behaviour to identify priorities due to coping and responding daily. Family resilience may be low due to personal circumstances and the length of time they have been managing with or without support. It is important to consider transference of behaviours and that decisions made now may affect behaviours in the future, particularly as children grow and become stronger.

An example

A child's play in the home was focused on a toy lawnmower. What happens when they outgrow it? A neighbour offers their old hover mower, providing the same enjoyment at a more suitable size. This offer is replicated by others... However, the old hover mowers are not intended for indoor use, causing damage to rooms and furniture, and end up 'taking over' the family room. Strange but true...

Hindsight tells us finding an alternative focus as they outgrew the toy would have made life easier.

Managing expectations

Parents and caregivers may be risk-averse, wanting to adapt all rooms, but it isn't practical to adapt a person's whole home environment. It is important to manage expectations from the beginning to ensure the best possible outcomes, promoting joint planning between professionals and families. For example, when a person likes water play and floods rooms, access to rooms can be restricted and mechanisms to prevent water access can be installed, but the person will still need to be able to bathe, so a balance is needed.

Associated outcomes

Costs and benefits of adaptations can be difficult to articulate, so you must evidence why you are making recommendations. Having the right environment will reduce the frequency or impact of behaviours that challenge, benefiting the person and those they live with, reducing stress and incidents resulting in damage to property. Altering environments also promotes socialization, facilitating ongoing relationships.

We know that annual costs for residential care are high. If an adaptation enables the person to remain at home, you could compare the cost of the adaptation with projected residential care fees. This demonstrates that although the budgets are separate, there are savings to the public purse. Preventing or reducing the severity of an injury and promoting good mental health has benefits for people as well as for associated health and social care systems and other agencies.

Sources of information

As an occupational therapist you will be approached to identify appropriate adaptations. But where do you get your information and advice from? Recommendations are underpinned by your initial assessment and observations, working in partnership with the individual, their parents and caregivers. It is useful to understand if behaviours occur in other settings – school, day centres or short break settings. This will support an understanding of the causes and management in these settings.

What do you do if you are struggling to find an appropriate solution? Colleagues may have seen and resolved something similar, assisting you through a discussion of options. That fresh pair of eyes can bring a new perspective as well as their prior experience.

Another source of support is the RCOT Specialist Section. If you are a member of the RCOT you will be able to approach them directly; if not, Twitter and other social media will enable you to make contact and call on their expertise. (See also the 'Useful resources' section at the end of the chapter.)

This is a developing area of practice, so the sources of support are growing. Publications such as *Designing Mind-Friendly Environments* (Maslin 2021), *Design for the Mind* (BSI 2022) and research papers all add to the evidence base.

Restrictive practices

It is imperative to consider the Mental Capacity Act (MCA) 2005, which applies to anyone over the age of 16. For those under 16, look at the principles listed below and consider the young person's views where possible; remember the challenge of removing practices introduced at an early age (consider the lawnmower scenario above).

Occupational therapists must:

- Balance safety and risk.

- Take reasonable steps to identify if the person does or doesn't have capacity to make an unwise decision.

- Consider if the person is deprived of their liberty.

- Identify the least restrictive option.

Restriction is not always physical. Safety concerns may result in increased oversight to minimize risks, but this is still a restrictive practice. Technology enables monitoring options including movement sensors, pressure pads, door alerts, video and audio monitors, and some options allow for two-way conversations. Increased availability and convenience of these devices is enhanced by the ability to link to phones and smart speakers. Where caregivers have concerns, increased levels of monitoring are understandable, but the MCA requires you to consider the implications.

Parental or caregiver oversight usually reduces as a child matures. When monitoring is retained it may become normalized and not recognized as a restriction. Be sure that consent to a practice is not simply because something has always been in place. There are times when oversight is appropriate, although this is based on individual need.

Sleep issues

As highlighted, some members of the person's household have reduced resilience from the effects of long-term behaviours that challenge. This is compounded by sleep deprivation due to the need for overnight monitoring for safety, and even more so if they have a disturbed sleep pattern. Lack of sleep affects health and wellbeing, and can reduce caregivers' ability to provide care and maintain employment, and for siblings, their education, with a reduced ability to concentrate at school.

The person may be at risk overnight due to their behaviours (e.g., eating non-edible objects (Pica), absconding, climbing or head banging) or they may be a risk to others (e.g., physical aggression including biting, hitting or inappropriate sexual behaviour).

Adaptations include alterations to the bedroom to encourage sleep or to reduce risks when the person is awake. Low-cost options, such as using white noise, altering light levels or using door locks to restrict access to items or rooms, should be trialled in the first instance. In the event of a sibling sharing a bedroom with the person, which places them at risk, adaptations may be considered to provide a separate sleeping space for the sibling, or alternatively, rehousing to a property with sufficient bedrooms may be a more suitable option.

Poor sleep patterns can have a significant impact, including:

- Parents preventing a young person leaving their bedroom at night by sleeping outside their door.

- Autistic siblings with differing sensory processing needs who are unable to share a bedroom without conflict, placing them at risk of injury.

Damage and destruction of property

Behaviours that challenge can be destructive to a property, which, in turn, may place the person or others at risk of injury. Here are some adaptation examples to reduce risk of damage:

- Toughened safety glass.

- Solid fire doors replacing hollow internal doors.

- Integral curtains or blinds.

- High-level heating systems installed or underfloor heating.

- Radiators and television enclosed with lockable doors.

- Wet room without a shower screen or curtain.

- Wipeable wall or floor covering.

Try to identify the cause of the destructive behaviour. It may relate to an uncomfortable sensory input such as the volume on a television, or alternatively, meeting sensory needs through compulsive repetitive behaviours such as banging on a pane of glass. Solutions will depend on the level of risk, identifying alternative ways of meeting the sensory needs of the person and the needs of others in the household.

Water, gas and electricity safety

Household utilities are essential, but are also potential hazards, with a risk of injury to people as well as damage to property. As always, identifying why a particular activity provides the feedback sought assists when considering how to divert attention or prevent a behaviour.

Sometimes it is necessary to prevent access to a facility. The easiest method may appear to be by locking the room, although this is not always practical, especially with facilities such as toilets where others need access. Locks can be used if all family members can manage them, but they are only effective if everyone remembers to use them. Any locks chosen need to be of a design or in a position that means the person with the challenging behaviour is unable to operate them. As always, any decision to use an adaptation that is restrictive needs to consider capacity, consent and the MCA.

Water

First, consider the issue:

- Is the basin being blocked by toilet paper because the person wants to splash in a bowl of water?

- Is the toilet flush handle frequently broken because they want to listen to running water?

- Is there a risk of scalding because they run the hot tap?

- Has there been flooding because taps are turned on and left?

The next step is to consider how to maintain access but minimize the issue. Suggestions include:

- Installing push handle taps that limit the flow of water.

- Changing the toilet flush mechanism to a push type.

- Fitting thermostatically controlled taps to minimize the risk of scalding.

- Removing plugs from basins and baths.

Gas

The risk of burns from gas hobs is high. Solutions to minimize risk include:

- Control knobs with safety covers installed to prevent them being operated.

- Fire guards can be used for fires.[1]

- Gas fires with remote control operation reduce risk.

- Radiators should have individual thermostats.

---

1   Fire or radiator guards intended for young children may not be robust enough to withstand challenging behaviours.

- Radiator covers can be installed securely fixed to a wall.

Electricity

Here the issue might be pulling down pendant light fittings, interfering with plug sockets or damage to light switches through repetitive use. Solutions include:

- Sensor lights if the issue is repetitive flicking on and off of a light switch.

- Downlighters installed, replacing pendant or wall lights.

- Lockable plug socket covers (similar to external socket covers used in the garden).[2]

- Limiting the use of extension cables and trailing wires for freestanding lights etc.

- Electric ovens can be switched off at the wall when not in use.

These are all direct actions, but sometimes a more indirect action is required, such as restricting the utility itself. Gas, water and electricity can all be restricted without affecting the whole property. Water isolation switches can be installed either adjacent to the basin, bath or toilet, or outside of the room. These are operated as you would a light switch, as you enter or leave a room, although there is a risk that over time this new action may become associated with access to water. Gas isolation switches can be located so the oven and hob can't be used, but if the issue is linked to the boiler, it may be more practical to enclose that in a lockable cupboard. Electrical circuits can be wired so they can be shut down when the person at risk is unsupervised, such as overnight. This maintains power to the majority of a home but ensures safety.

Risks are not always directly linked to the utility but to the equipment utilizing it, for example a shower. Shower hoses can be a ligature risk or the unit can be pulled from the wall. Ligature risk can be removed by installing a rainfall shower head plumbed in from the ceiling. Installing shower control units outside of the shower area provides access to bathing so caregivers can regulate the temperature and flow of water, maintaining safety and supporting privacy and dignity during bathing.

---

2   Plug-in safety covers are not recommended, as the socket is live when they are inserted, and may be a choke hazard.

Compulsion to eat

Some people with conditions such as Pica or Prader-Willi syndrome seek out edible and non-edible items and can ingest unsafe solids or liquids or eat to excess. Pica is a drive or need to eat non-food items. With Pica the compulsion to eat items with no nutritional value varies between people, so a person-centred approach is key, and a resolution may take time to identify. Those with Prader-Willi syndrome often develop a compulsion to eat, which becomes a behaviour that challenges when it cannot be managed through monitoring, diversion or persuasion. There is a hazard to health from gastric issues, poisoning or health issues associated with overeating or a poor diet.

Limiting access to food items may be resolved through lockable cupboards, including preventing access to the kitchen bin or the dishwasher. Non-food items that should be locked away include cleaning fluids and bathroom items such as shower gel, toothpaste and cosmetics. Overnight it may be that just the kitchen door needs to be secured, as usually bathroom access needs to be maintained for others.

Adaptations to reduce the risks associated with this can require lateral thinking. For example:

- Cladding walls with acrylic panels or vinyl flooring prevents access to wall plaster.

- Changing floor coverings from carpet to laminate or vinyl works, but the fitting needs to be secure and tight to the walls.

- Fuse boxes with a residual-current device (RCD) breaker should be installed.

- Additional RCD breakers can be used in areas where cables can be nibbled.

- Avoid fixtures and fittings with removable parts, such as rubber bungs, including thermostats and controls.

De-escalation spaces

People displaying behaviours that challenge often benefit from a calm environment with reduced stimuli to de-escalate. However, there are potential disadvantages to evaluate when considering a specific location for a de-escalation space (whether this is a room, tent or 'safe space').

It isn't practical in a home for the whole environment to remain in a consistent calming condition; family life has to continue. Calming physical features may be difficult to identify if it feels like nothing works. It may be that the person is unable to self-identify when they will benefit from accessing a calming space, or they become overstimulated in another location.

How can they be encouraged to relocate? It isn't appropriate to manually lift or manhandle them, and they are less likely to rationalize a need to relocate. They may also respond aggressively. The person could become socially isolated through choosing to spend time in the de-escalation space or through being placed there. They may be habituated to this environment and find it more difficult to regulate their behaviour in other environments. In evaluating a need for a de-escalation space, consider the MCA, Deprivation of Liberty Safeguards (DoLS) and the risk of neglect or social isolation.

Access and exit points

Doors and windows serve a number of purposes: access, ventilation and to ensure safety and home security, but for some, a response over and above daily home security is needed. The challenge is to ensure that the minimum level of restriction is applied. MCA requirements mean that although securing a door or window may seem sensible, we cannot simply recommend this. Always ask yourself, 'Is this typical for a person of this age?' If the answer is no, consider processes to ensure the least restrictive option is employed.

Doors

Where access to a room needs to be limited, a stable or Dutch door can be installed, often replacing a stair gate. These are divided horizontally, either at the mid-point or at two-thirds height. How and when this is secured to prevent access to or from the room will require a risk evaluation, as it is restrictive.

Glazed viewing panels or 360° viewers can be used to enable oversight without opening the door, but as these are not typically used within a home, they are considered a restrictive practice. Again, a risk evaluation will evidence your professional reasoning supporting this recommendation.

Altering handles on doors may prevent someone leaving the room or accessing other rooms. This includes installing dual handles or a door knob rather than lever handles for someone who has difficulty in using this handle design. Where this is used to prevent freedom of movement rather than safety – you guessed right – this is a restriction!

Locks

Sometimes something simple like a star lock or a bolt can be enough to ensure safety.

Technology means that locks can be operated by apps rather than keys, but they still fall within the MCA remit. If a lock is added to prevent access or leaving a room, be clear why you are recommending this and for what benefit. (It may seem counterintuitive, but if a household member is at risk from a person who exhibits challenging behaviour, a lock may be an appropriate solution. If the person at risk is able to operate a lock and has capacity to consent to its use, then providing them with a way of securing their door for their safety may be the right action. This would not be our first line of thought, but one to consider.)

> For any locking system used, liaison with the Fire and Rescue Service is advised so in the event of an incident they are aware of additional barriers to access.

Windows/ventilation/sills

Windows can increase risk if a person lacks risk awareness, both as an exit point and due to glazing. Additional or alternative locks can be used, but this, in itself, raises issues around ventilation; mechanical ventilation can be installed but may create background noise. An alternative is to create a barrier that enables a window to be opened safely. Clear perforated Perspex, vinyl or similar on an internal frame can enable a window to be used...but for some this barrier may provide a focus for sensory feedback.

Usually, fire escape windows will not have locks fitted, but Building Regulations (HM Government 2016) do allow for these to be installed. If the issue is climbing on the window sill, then installing a sloped insert removes the option to climb.

Glazing

Safety film can be applied, reducing risk if glass is broken, but it is always sensible to ensure glazing is toughened glass in areas where someone is unsupervised.

Issues around glazing aren't only associated with breakage or injury. Where a person prefers not to wear clothes or does not moderate their behaviour in line with social norms, windows means they are visible to members of the public. Minimizing the impact of this may require integral blinds, set between the two panes of double glazing, applying a film to obscure the glass (possibly on the external pane to prevent removal) or installing obscured glass.

Lighting and control of light levels

Lighting is a potential source for behaviours that challenge, including continuously flicking switches on and off, pulling light bulbs or fittings and playing with the wire, or the impact of sensory-processing difficulties relating to vision and light. These behaviours are unlikely to present or require adaptations on their own, but rather form part of the bigger picture. Consider:

- Switches outside of the bedroom/out of reach/voice-activated.

- Flush lighting (no lamps or hanging cords).

- Integral blinds/Velcro curtains.

- Coloured bulbs.

- Dimmer switches.

Room padding vs. 'safe spaces'

Where there is a risk of self-injury through interactions with walls or radiators, then padding a room is an option. The benefit of this is that the person is protected, but there are downsides to consider. First, this is only one space, and risks remain elsewhere. Second, what needs to be padded? All, or just part, of the room? Is there a need for a specific area to be made safe, such as around the bed or over a radiator? What happens if part of the padding is damaged? Responsibility for repairs or replacements is important, as a single section can be costly to replace. (If the padding is provided via a DFG, then responsibility to fund repairs or a replacement lies with the person or their family.)

A padded adult-size cot bed may be appropriate, but provides less choice and freedom than a bed within a padded room. Cot beds can provide the benefits of a height-adjustable platform, supporting caregivers in managing personal care. This resolves the issues within the bed space, but not in the wider area.

There are robustly constructed 'safe space' structures that can be erected inside a room. These also limit a person's choice and freedom, but have the advantage that they can be relocated if a person moves properties. There is a debate around funding in some areas, however, as they may not be considered an adaptation. Assessing and understanding sensory processing and personal preferences will enable you to evaluate if this is an appropriate method of meeting need. Having an enclosed space within a room may provide the option for a caregiver to monitor the person, and allows items like televisions and sensory equipment to be protected. The alternative is that these are housed behind safety screens as part of an adaptation.

Because of the enclosed nature of all these options, ventilation is key. Cot beds and 'safe spaces' may allow for windows to be left open, but they have reduced airflow within the enclosure. If a room needs to be fully padded, then the windows are often protected with perforated vinyl or Perspex screens, which have the same effect.

Remember for all the suggested options that the MCA, DoLs and Liberty Protection Safeguards (LPS) must be considered...a full assessment and risk evaluation must be followed to evidence why this is the most appropriate option.

Smearing

People displaying behaviours that challenge may have a learning disability and reduced capacity to care for themselves independently. This will include maintaining their personal hygiene. Smearing of faeces is a behaviour that can be particularly challenging to family and caregivers, and particularly if it is linked with Pica. Efforts should be made in the first instance to determine why the person is smearing. Do they like the smell? Are they seeking the texture? Are they compelled to eat, or do they like the taste? Can other opportunities be provided to meet this sensory need to reduce the risk of smearing happening in the first instance?

People may wear continence products and can gain access to the contents. 'Houdini' suits can be a method of preventing access but are restrictive and people can often find a way to get into them. Surfaces including furniture, walls and floors should be wipe-clean, where possible, to reduce staining and offensive odours. This includes access routes to the bathroom, and it may be that you need to limit access to other areas of the environment to prevent contamination. This can be especially challenging in homes where the bathroom is accessed via the kitchen.

Adaptations to reduce the impact of behaviours that challenge extend outside of the building to include the garden area (see Chapter 19 for information on adapting outdoor spaces).

Identifying the causes of a behaviour can be a challenge. This is an area of occupational therapy practice where collaboration and multi-disciplinary working will enable you to reduce the impact of behaviours and to promote the resilience of family members.

Useful resources

- *DLF factsheets*: https://livingmadeeasy.org.uk/dlf-factsheets

- *Foundations*: www.foundations.uk.com

- *The Challenging Behaviour Foundation*: www.challenging behaviour.org.uk

(If you use an online forum, please ensure that all information is anonymized.)

18

Enabling Mobility and Access

Knowledge check

* What is the difference between 'clear' and 'effective' opening door widths?

* What is the difference between a grab rail and a handrail?

* How many different types of door can you think of that are found in a domestic dwelling?

* What gradient should a ramp be?

Adaptations promote ease of entering and exiting the home, but also the ability to move around the home and access essential facilities. Here we look at adaptations individually, but in reality these are used in combination to ensure that those you are supporting can access essential facilities and live the lives they choose.

Doors

Doorways provide us with the ability to enter and use our home, to exit and access communities, providing educational, employment and leisure opportunities. This approach already conveys that a door is more than something filling a gap in a wall.

The doorway has a number of aspects to consider. You must understand the structure of a door to appreciate aspects you will be reviewing to ensure it is usable and suitable for the person:

* *Structural opening:* This is the space doors are set into. On architectural

drawings a gap in a wall may be indicated. You need to understand if this is the structural opening or the door set (see below). The size of the structural opening dictates the usable space left when the doorway is complete.

- *Door set:* This is everything – frame, door, handles etc. Some schemes will specify a door set while others provide the size of the door itself.

- *Casing:* This is the door frame on which the door is hung. The size of this within the structural opening affects the size of the opening available.

- *Door leaf:* This is the door. It may be solid, part-glazed, fully glazed, a fire door…there are numerous options.

- *Hinge and lock side:* Pretty obvious, but worth mentioning, a door is attached to the frame (hung) by the hinge side. Viewing architectural drawings in plan view reduces errors that might occur if you are discussing options in a vertical plane, as you could be viewing the doorway from different rooms.

- *Hinges:* The method by which the door is hung from the frame. There are various types and designs. Typically hinges allow for the door to open to at least 90°. Parliament hinges enable the door leaf to open flat against a wall, providing a wider opening, and 180° hinges allow for a door leaf to open in either direction (there won't be a door stop installed in the frame for this option), and loose pin hinges enable access in an emergency for inward-opening doors. (Sliding door designs don't have hinges, but will be hung from a track.)

- *Door stop:* These prevent over-swing of the door, and although they are quite slim, they add to the reduction of space available to pass through the doorway.

- *Door furniture:* Anything added to a door – handles, locks, door knockers. If they stand proud of the door they will reduce the space to pass through the opening.

- *Clear opening width:* This is how far the door opens to give the space between the door and the frame on the lock side.

- *Effective opening width:* This is the usable space you are left with when you take into account all of the above, and is actually the space that matters most!

Watch the video 'The anatomy of a door' (3 minutes 26 seconds) at https://library.jkp.com/redeem, using the code EDKQQWA.

Knowledge check

Look at Figure 20. What type of door is adjacent to the numbers and/or why do you think this has been highlighted? A larger image is available at https://library.jkp.com/redeem (using the code EDKQQWA), and the answers are given at the end of this chapter.

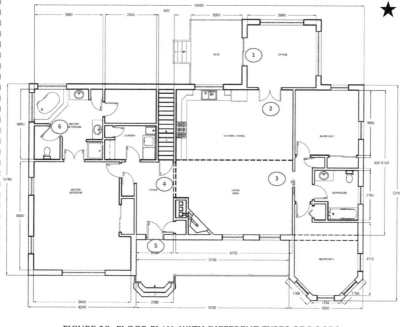

FIGURE 20. FLOOR PLAN, WITH DIFFERENT TYPES OF DOORS
Source: Andrea Cox

Doors and doorways

Level thresholds facilitate accessibility at doorways. Usually, internal doorways are level, but there can be changes in level caused by different floor coverings, either joining strips or the addition of multiple flooring layers in one room. Ideally external doors will have level thresholds, but this is a relatively new requirement. Low thresholds still present barriers to wheelchair users, albeit less than the thresholds on uPVC and composite door sets.

Grab rails

Grab rails are available in several sizes, the most common being 300mm, 450mm and 600mm, with a choice of grips and colours. When considering the placement, size and orientation of a grab rail, it is important to identify who is using the grab rail, what purpose it serves and where it is being used.

Grab rails are a cost-effective adaptation and can make a significant difference for the individual they have been prescribed for. However, there is an inherent danger that grab rails can be overprescribed, and almost used as a catch-all solution on steps and stairs.

Where are grab rails best situated?

Changes in floor level

Grab rails can be effectively used to support transition between floor levels. At single steps such as between a sitting room and kitchen you may want to consider a smaller grab rail. When prescribing a grab rail consider:

- Placement of the grab rail.

- Height above the step nosing or from the lowest floor level.

- Door width.

- Mobility aids.

- Visual impairment.

- Diagnosis or disability.

On steps and at door thresholds

Are the steps internal or external? What orientation of the rail is appropriate? A longer rail can be orientated in different planes. Figures 21a–c illustrate three options. A vertical installation (Figure 21a) offers support on approach or exit, a horizontal installation (Figure 21b) balance on stepping up or down. A diagonal rail (Figure 21c) the length of a flight of steps offers continuous support as the change of level is negotiated.

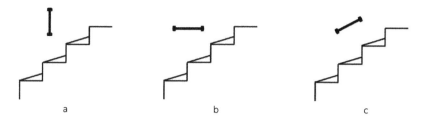

FIGURES 21A–C. GRAB RAILS ADJACENT TO STEPS
Source: David Owen and Ruth Parker

Near or adjacent to a toilet

Why is the grab rail needed? Does it support a lateral transfer for a wheelchair user? Is it supporting a sit-to-stand transfer, or is it to support somebody to stand and use the toilet? See Figures 22a–e.

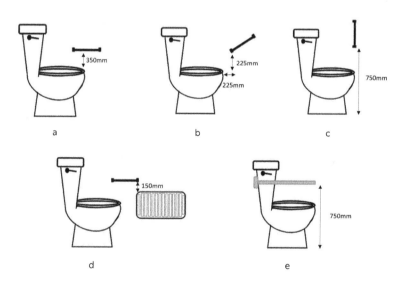

FIGURES 22A–E. GRAB RAILS ADJACENT TO A TOILET
Source: David Owen and Ruth Parker

HORIZONTAL RAIL

Lateral transfers benefit from a longer grab rail set above the toilet pan approximately between 200mm and 350mm (see Figure 22a). The grab rail is positioned with the centre point aligned to the pan edge. The benefit of this is that the grab rail can help with transfers and movements while sitting on the toilet, such as reaching to cleanse after toileting.

DIAGONAL RAIL IN FORWARD REACH POSITION

A diagonal rail set in front and slightly above the toilet pan supports sit-to-stand transfers as it encourages the individual to reach forward as they stand, and it may help with balance while cleansing after using the toilet (see Figure 22b).

VERTICAL RAIL IN FORWARD REACH POSITION

This layout may be useful for a person who is able to stand with minimal difficulty but who requires support in transition into standing, and to steady themselves before walking away (see Figure 22c).

HORIZONTAL GRAB RAIL ABOVE A RADIATOR

This layout is useful when a radiator is positioned next to the toilet to prevent the use of the radiator for support (see Figure 22d). Potential risks here are evident:

- A burn due to a high radiator temperature.

- The radiator being pulled away from the wall due to increased pressure being placed on wall fixings.

- A fall, as the radiator is not designed to support a person.

WALL OR FLOOR-MOUNTED DROP-DOWN RAIL

This layout is useful where a lateral transfer is used or equipment space is limited. The rail can be raised when not in use and lowered when needed; these rails can be used for support when adjusting position on the toilet and raised for cleansing after toileting (see Figure 22e).

For those who require a greater level of support, options with a supporting leg are available. Of course, the above can be used in combination if required.

Around the bath or shower

Similar to rails adjacent to the toilet, rail configuration will support the needs of different users. Figures 23, 24 and 25 illustrate positions where grab rails can be useful in promoting safe access to bathing. Your holistic person-centred assessment will guide you on the ideal position for rails reflecting their movement pattern and transfer abilities.

HORIZONTAL RAIL ABOVE THE BATH

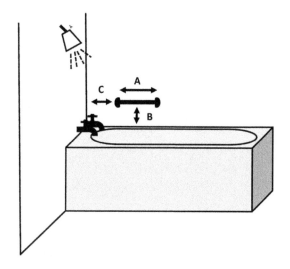

FIGURE 23. HORIZONTAL GRAB RAIL ABOVE THE BATH
Source: Ruth Parker and David Owen

DIAGONAL RAIL ABOVE THE BATH

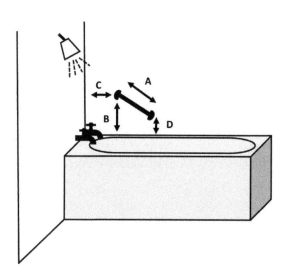

FIGURE 24. DIAGONAL GRAB RAIL ABOVE THE BATH
Source: Ruth Parker and David Owen

VERTICAL RAIL ABOVE THE BATH

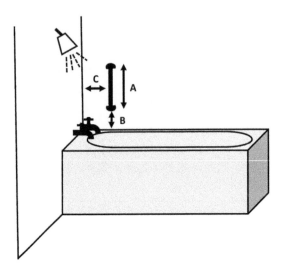

FIGURE 25. VERTICAL GRAB RAIL ABOVE THE BATH
Source: Ruth Parker and David Owen

Handrails

What is the difference between a grab rail and a handrail? Grab rails are provided in designated lengths, and a handrail is a continuous length or rail to span defined points.

Where are handrails best situated?

Handrails can be useful where an individual needs to travel over a slightly longer distance, for example a set of stairs, corridor, graded pathway or a ramp. The choice and position of the handrail will depend on what function it needs to perform as well as location – indoors or outdoors.

Construction

The material you specify will depend on where the handrail is located. You will usually encounter two materials:

- *Wood:* Appropriate for use indoors; this may be installed outdoors but requires maintenance and has reduced longevity.

- *Galvanized metal:* Usually used outdoors as it is corrosion-resistant.

Shape

Handrails come in a variety of shapes, some of which are easier to use. The most ergonomic design is a 50mm diameter circular rail (*mopstick*) with a flat edge at the base providing mounting points for fixings. The *pig's ear* design offer a less secure grip, and is not usually recommended as part of an adaptation. *Exterior* rails are usually circular, with a 50mm diameter.

When negotiating corners, generally speaking, where a handrail follows a corner it should be continuous so the user does not have to remove their hand, especially on stairs.

Stairs

Stairs can present a challenge for users as there is a wide variety of stair shapes and designs. Buildsafe provides some useful information related to stair regulations in the UK.[1]

Knowledge check

What are the different parts of a staircase called? (Answers are provided at the end of this chapter.)

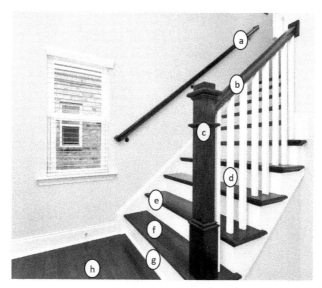

FIGURE 26. PARTS OF A STAIRCASE

---

1   https://buildsafe.co.uk/stair-regulations-in-the-uk

Layout

Stairs will either be an *open* design where you are able to see through the stair riser or *closed* with a solid riser. These are the most common types of layouts you are likely to encounter:

- *Straight:* A straight flight of stairs is simply that, they lead in a direct line between the adjoining floors.

- *Top winder:* This type of staircase generally has a straight section leading from the lower floor and then a curved section of stairs typically around three stairs as it reaches the upper floor. The curved sections of stairs are wider on one side.

- *Bottom winder:* This layout is the opposite of the top winder, where the curve is on the lower floor and the straight section leads to the upper floor level.

- *Dog-legged:* This type of staircase usually has two straight sections that run in contrary directions and are separated by a half or two-quarter landing. In cases where there are two-quarter landings there may be one stair separating each of the landings.

- *Spiral:* A spiral staircase usually has a continual double curve, similar to a double helix.

- *Middle winder:* This layout of staircase generally has two straight sections, one leading from the lower level and the other leading from the upper floor level connected with a curved section of stairs.

Width

The width of the stairs is important as this can determine if one or two handrails can be fitted and if a stairlift can be accommodated. Also bear in mind the stature of the person, as this will affect adaptation options.

Tread depth (or going)

Tread depth is important: if the person is not able to place their foot wholly on each stair, there is an increased risk of falls.

Space at the top and bottom of the stairs

Space at the top and bottom of the stairs is important as this facilitates a safe transition from the stairs to the floor level. Obstructions or lack of space here make the transition from stairs to the floor difficult and pose a risk of falls. The person may reach out to furniture or other objects when completing this transition, and so it is sensible to keep these areas clear of obstructions, especially if a walking aid is used. The person may require the use of a walking aid on each floor level, and obstructions may impede its use. This advice extends to all areas of the stairs including half-landings. Grab rails in transition areas may be helpful with increasing safety.

Some questions to consider are:

- Are these areas free of obstruction?

- Can grab rails be fitted to aid negotiation?

- Is there sufficient space for a stairlift transfer area?

Lighting

Effective lighting is essential on any staircase, whether it is internal or external. As we age our visual acuity decreases and poor lighting may contribute to trips and falls. Another factor to consider around lighting is how the lighting source is activated. Can it be activated before the ascent or descent of the stairs? Is the light source sufficient to illuminate the whole staircase?

Floor covering

The floor covering of stairs is important in terms of providing a firm base for feet to gain traction, enabling transition from stair to stair. The first factor to consider is actually the footwear that the individual wears:

- Do they wear a sturdy shoe with a rubber sole that provides good grip?

- Do they wear socks indoors?

- Do their socks have grips on the sole?

- Do they walk around barefoot?

The type of floor covering, such as carpet, painted wood or bare wood, impacts on the ability to gain traction and may influence the type of footwear that is used or recommended. For example, if the floor covering is carpet, then wearing socks may offer sufficient grip to the foot. Alternatively wood treads offer little grip, and rubber-soled footwear should be recommended.

The quality and fitting of the floor covering is important, especially on the stair nosing and in the riser corner. If the covering is poorly fitted or worn, this increases risk. Some questions to consider are:

- Does the stair covering offer sufficient slip-resistance for the user, considering their footwear preference?

- Is the floor covering securely fitted to the stairs on the stair nosing and at the riser corner?

Stair rails

Stair rails are an essential safety item to support and encourage safe use of the stairs. Current Building Regulations (HM Government 2016) require at least one rail on a staircase under 1000mm wide. When thinking about the type of handrail it is important to consider the width of the stairs, the staircase pitch and the person's height, grip and upper body strength. When measuring and prescribing a stair rail, start with the person standing, with their arms relaxed at their side. Then measure from the floor to their wrist.

Considerations for prescription of a stair rail include:

- When specifying the handrail height, the measurement given is from *nosing to the required height.*

- Describing the installation position, it is given as left- or right-side *ascending.*

- Advise if there are curves or corners on the stairs and that the handrail must be continuous.

- Where possible the stair rail should extend beyond the top and bottom step to support transition.

- Another area to consider is a turn in the stairs and how you might provide support on a turn.

Here are some other questions to consider:

- Are there stair rails in place?

- Do they extend the whole length of the staircase?

- Are there any turns in the stairs that require the user to take their hand off a handrail?

External stairs

The principles of external stairs are similar to those of internal stairs, although there are some important differences. External stairs may either be covered or open to the elements, and may be constructed from a range of materials, including wood, metal or concrete. If the stairs are covered or partially covered, this is likely to increase safety and ease of use. However, stairs that are open to the elements increase potential risk as the stairs are subject to water ingress, freezing and collection of debris, increasing the risk of trips and slips.

The tread surface of external stairs is likely to be a hard surface and should have a slip-resistant finish. In some cases, the tread surface will have a low traction finish that could lead to reduced grip. External stairs can provide access to multiple dwellings and must meet relevant standards. This can present a challenge when adapting for an individual.

Steps

There are universal considerations for steps (internal and external). First, consider the person:

- How do they mobilize?

- Do they use any mobility aids?

- Do they have any sensory impairments?

- Are there cognitive impairments to consider?

Second, consider the steps themselves:

- Where do they lead?

- What is the step width?

- Tread depth?

- Riser height?

- Surface finish?

Let's look at external steps. When adapting steps, it's important to look at where they lead and their state of repair. For example, if there are two steps leading from a rear doorway to a level area and the steps are in a good state of repair, a handrail may be sufficient.

What about a more complex case, with two steps leading to a front door and the person walks with the aid of a walking frame? A handrail would not be sufficient and the steps themselves may need adapting. In this instance you may need to increase the tread depth and step width and reduce the rise of each step. This may increase the overall number of steps. Another aspect to consider is, does the person require carer support? This will impact on your decision on the size and shape of the steps needed. You may also consider whether a ramp would be a better solution.

In some circumstances a ramp is less desirable as it may increase the distance the person walks and make using a ramp unfeasible. It may be better to have steps with deep treads and a low rise, as this will allow the person to negotiate each step and rest while covering a shorter distance. This decision is supported by your assessment and observations.

Handrails are an important consideration on steps, with the height, position, choice of material and finish of the handrail tailored to the person.

The surface finish of steps will depend on whether the steps are a new construction or are being adapted. The surface finish should generally be slip-resistant; this could be a brushed concrete finish, paving stones, slip-resistant strips or a covering of a slip-resistant paint. Slip-resistant strips and paint are less desirable, however, as they are prone to wear and require maintenance.

Another aspect to consider is how the user identifies the edge of the step, especially where they have a visual impairment. Avoid a step that has a significant overhang as this is a trip hazard. Also consider a colour-contrasting finish to the step and nosing. Highlighting the nosing with white or yellow paint is effective.

Ramps

Considerations for installing a ramp include the person and the start and end points of a ramp. First, mobility: how does the person mobilize? Do they walk with a walking aid, or with a walking aid and the support of another? Do they use a self-propelling wheelchair or attendant-propelled wheelchair? Or do they have a powered wheelchair that is self-controlled or attendant-controlled? Also consider the size of the wheelchair when establishing the minimum size of landing areas and turns. Ultimately, responsibility for creating a suitable scheme lies with the designer, but they need this information, and, as the prescriber, you need to be aware of any ramp limitations.

Next, consider the ramp design and general specifications. There are several schools of thought when prescribing a ramp adaptation. Do you provide a highly detailed specification or a description of what is required? For example, 'Person A uses a manual wheelchair of X dimension and requires wheelchair or step-free access between the property and street level'. This approach leaves interpretation of what is to be provided to the scheme designer.

Consider the physical characteristics of the ramp:

- *Gradient:* This refers to the steepness of the ramp. Generally speaking, the steeper the ramp, the harder it is for the person to use. **Part M of**

the Building Regulations recommends the steepest usable gradient is a ratio of 1:12 – every inch of height needed equates to 12 inches of ramp distance (HM Government 2016).

- *Width:* Think of this in two ways – the overall width of a ramp and unobstructed width (or usable space). It is recommended that ramps have an overall width of 1200mm and an unobstructed width of 1000mm.

- *Length:* Ramp length is an important consideration. The height difference between the start and end of the ramp determines both length and usability. For example, a 10m-long ramp may suit a powered wheelchair user but pose a significant challenge to a self-propelling wheelchair user.

- *Upstands:* These prevent mobility aids from going over the edge of the ramp. They are usually 100mm in height and vary in construction material.

- *Handrails:* Where the height difference between a ramp and adjacent ground level is greater than 600mm, handrails must be provided. The next question is: should the handrail be a single or double rail? Some wheelchair services require a double rail to further reduce the risk of a wheelchair going over the edge of a ramp. Consider both the person and wheelchair type. For young children in self-propelled wheelchairs a double rail handrail is essential.

- *Surface finish:* This depends on the ramp construction. Those constructed from concrete could have a brushed surface finish, while metal ramps may have a rubberized or other type of slip-resistant finish.

- *Permanent or semi-permanent:* There is a debate over these options. There are now cost-effective modular ramp systems providing a timely and reusable solution. The obvious benefits of semi-permanent solutions are that they can be installed quickly, they avoid the need for significant construction, and can be reused or resited.

- *Start/end points:* Where does the ramp start and finish? You would expect the start and end point of the ramp to have a suitable circulation space for the wheelchair or mobility aid being used. Aim for a landing area of around 1000 x 1000mm, 1200 x 1200mm, 1500 x 1500mm or 1800 x 1800mm. This is, of course, dependent on the space available at the desired location as well as the user's needs.

- *Property exit/entry point:* How does the person exit and enter the dwelling? In which direction does the door open? Outward opening requires more space to accommodate the door-opening arc. Other adaptations to the exit/entry point of the property may be required, including door widening, change of threshold, powered door opener and door entry system.

- *Landing size/position:* Part M of the Building Regulations (HM Government 2016) requires level platforms at set distances for longer ramps. This may result in a ramp that has a number of returns.

Also consider: *is a ramp the best option?* And are there any other options such as external lifts or inclined platform lifts?

Lighting on external access adaptations (ramps, pathways, steps and stairs)

The issues presented around lighting can be complex and contentious. From a person-centred perspective, the provision of suitable lighting enabling access is often overlooked. This can have a significant impact on how and when the person can use the adaptation provided for them. Where a person has a visual impairment, provision of suitable lighting can be universally reasoned.

Issues arise where there isn't a sensory impairment. Ultimately decisions around the inclusion of lighting as part of your recommendation will depend on the functional need, including when and how an adaptation will be used. Where does the adaptation for access start and lead to? Where it leads from a main access point to street level and is provided to ensure the individual can access the community, considerations include:

- Is there sufficient street lighting within a reasonable distance from the property?

- Does street lighting allow the person to find their keys and insert them into the door lock?

- Does it provide sufficient lighting to identify any trip hazards?

- Does the individual regularly enter and exit their property during darkness?

- Does the adaptation design make it difficult to use in low light levels?

- Are other solutions available, such as the individual purchasing solar-powered lights?

- Is lighting needed to perform a specific task(s) to facilitate entry and exit to the property?

The point around a person entering and exiting their property during darkness hours is somewhat erroneous, which may be highlighted by an adaptation specifier: adaptations are prescribed to enable an individual to overcome an occupational barrier to participation. Therefore, you cannot suggest that they can only use the adaptation during daylight hours. You have to enable choice and control over when an individual chooses to enter and exit their home.

If the adaptation for access leads to a garden or drying area etc., then provision of lighting may be included in a recommendation if justified. However, consider if it is reasonable to advise that they should only use the space during daylight hours or that the person purchases solar lighting.

The argument for providing lighting to the main entry and exit route from the property to street level is stronger, as the person will need the ability to leave and return from their home at any point of the day. Social activities, work, domestic errands or a myriad of other reasons mean that entry and exit may be during low light levels, or at night, especially during winter months. This aligns with your role to enable people to overcome occupational barriers and participate in occupations of choice and necessity.

Stairlifts

Stairlifts are valuable adaptations that enable access between different floors in a person's home, but, importantly, also access to existing essential facilities. Stairlifts are available in two types – internal and external – and considerations for prescription are similar. If the person has a complex condition or the stairs have a complex layout, it would be prudent to be present on the survey visit.

Here are some aspects to consider when recommending a stairlift.

For the person:

- *Their stature:* Consider the person's height, weight and body shape.

Weight is important as stairlifts have safe working loads – typically 19 stone, 25 stone and in some cases, 30 stone.

- *Sitting ability:* Can they maintain a sitting position for the time it takes the stairlift to ascend or descend the stairs? Can they hold their feet on the footplate for that time?

- *Transfer ability:* How does the person transfer? Do they use a walking aid or are they a wheelchair user? Available space at the foot and top of the stairs will affect use.

- *Cognitive ability:* Does the person have the capacity to learn how to operate the stairlift? Do they need supervision? Assessment of executive function has demonstrated that stairlift use by those with dementia can be appropriate (Chung *et al.* 2018).

- *Dexterity:* Medical conditions or disability can limit dexterity and ability to operate controls.

- *Sensory impairments:* Visual impairment may impact safe transfers as well as actual stairlift use.

- *Contraindications:* Conditions causing absence seizures, involuntary body movements or freezing episodes may mean that use of a stairlift is inappropriate.

For the stairlift itself:

- *Location:* Internal or external.

- *Stairs:* Shape, layout, width and transfer areas.

- *Safe working load.*

- *Control type:* Joystick, paddle or button, position left and right or both.

- *Seat:* Standard or specialist for a child.

- *Seat mechanism:* Manual or powered.

- *Footplate:* Manual, powered or interlinked with seat.

- *Seatbelt:* Lap strap or harness.

- *Track:* Straight, curved, folding track, internal or external angle; does a hinged end section cover any part of a doorway when lowered? Does this affect access?

- *Location of parking position:* Bottom, top or partway up the stairs.

- *Reset switch* or key control location.

- *Audible/visual warnings.*

- *Servicing/repairs:* Who is responsible?

Through floor lift or platform lift

As with stairlifts, there are considerations to take into account when recommending a lift installation. These can be major installations requiring structural alterations and changes to room use. This solution can feel daunting to those being supported, but installation can restore access to all areas of the home and minimize risks associated with stair use. Here are some aspects to consider.

For the person:

- *Their stature:* Consider the person's height, weight and body shape. Weight is important as lifts have safe working loads (including any mobility or other equipment).

- *Ability to stand* or sit as the lift transitions between floors.

- *Ability to transfer* in/out of the lift or on/off the platform.

- *Mobility aids used,* such as a wheelchair, and its size and method of locomotion (self-propelled, powered, attendant-controlled etc.).

- *Cognitive ability:* Does the person have the capacity to learn how to operate the lift? Do they need supervision?

- *Dexterity:* The ability to operate controls. Medical conditions or disability can limit dexterity and ability to operate controls.

- *Sensory impairments:* Visual impairment may impact safe transfers as well as lift use.

- *Contraindications:* Conditions causing absence seizures, involuntary body movements, or freezing episodes may mean that use of a lift is inappropriate.

- *User supervision:* Does the person require direct supervision? This may impact the size and shape of the lift that may be required.

For the lift:

- *Location* of the lift: Is this to be situated within the property or is an external lift shaft to be created?

- *Position of the lift on each floor:* Are there any obstructions, or is a change in room use needed?

- *Size of lift:* To facilitate standing, seated or wheelchair use. Will it need to facilitate use by the person with their carer?

- *Space for door to open:* Again, consider any obstructions on each landing level.

- *Mechanism of door operation:* Whether manual or automatic operation, can the person operate the door, or does it need to be operated by another person?

- *Control type/mechanism:* Typically the controls of a lift and stairlift require the person to apply constant pressure to ensure the lift motion is continuous; if pressure is released, the lift will stop.

- *Does the person* use it independently/assisted/controlled by an attendant outside the lift/attendant inside the lift?

- *Type of car:* Open car or closed, or one that fits into a corner.

- *Lift shaft:* It may not always be possible to fit a lift with tracks, and a lift shaft will be required; these can be expensive and difficult to accommodate within a domestic setting. For an external lift a lift shaft may be necessary due to the terrain or surface conditions.

- *Steps:* Is an incline platform lift appropriate?

Supporting those with mobility impairments through home adaptations is possibly the area of occupational therapy with the greatest impact on those we support. Mobility impairments require a wide range of solutions, each tailored to the individual and their home environment. From low-cost solutions such as grab rails to major environmental changes, occupational therapists facilitate meaningful occupations, enable access to communities and support a person to make full use of their home environment.

Plan view of different types of doors (see Figure 20):

1. Sliding doors (external, leading to a decked area)

2. Internal double doors (hinged)

3. Pocket door

4. Single-leaf door at the foot of the stairs (likely to be a fire door)

5. External single-leaf door

6. Single-leaf internal door (setting it at an angle provides additional space in the room)

Parts of a staircase (see Figure 26):

(a) Stair or handrail; these are attached to a wall

(b) Bannister; these are rails supported by stair rods or balusters

(c) Newel post

(d) Stair rod or baluster

(e) Nosing

(f) Tread depth (or going)

(g) Riser

(h) Landing

19

Promoting Access to Outdoor Spaces

Knowledge check

* Who is responsible for agreeing to a dropped kerb?

* When must a pathway have an upstand?

* What is biophilia?

* Can provision of a driveway be restricted to full-time wheelchair users only?

* What is a TPO?

What do we mean by 'outside space'?

In this context, 'outside space' is the space around the home property that the occupant or owner has the ability to alter. In very general terms, this is the front garden, driveway and rear garden. As with everything, however, it is not as simple as that. Although these are used as the main ways of describing the area surrounding a property, not everyone has this 'typical' dwelling.

Some people live in flats with communal spaces or balconies; some with gardens that are not directly accessed from their home; and some don't have outside space at all. The outside space for someone who lives in a houseboat is quite different to a three-bedroomed semi-detached house on a new development. Your challenge is to promote access and occupations in whatever area is available to a person. You will need to understand what space is available, what control the person has over changes that may need to be made, and how the space is used.

This chapter looks at wider spaces and should be read in conjunction with Chapter 18.

Your assessment will provide you with an idea of how much a person and their household utilize available outdoor space. How we use our personal space differs, so you will need to return to the assessment to understand what it is that you are promoting. You may be a keen gardener or always hang your washing out on fine days, but this may not be what the person you are working with wants. They may want to have the ability to stand on their front doorstep to watch the world go by, or to have a cigarette. It doesn't matter what you consider to be appropriate; this is their space, and you must respect that. Although there will be times where you advise that an activity is not appropriate or safe, consider alternative ways in which this can be achieved.

A key question when considering outside space is, 'who is the space for?' This reflects the household and includes aspects such as pets and frequent visitors. In an ideal world you would support access for all, but you must take a pragmatic view. It would be lovely to support the annual visit of a frail elderly relative, but this is not appropriate or within most occupational therapy remits. On the other hand, if a person is able to fund the changes needed and wishes to do so, then you should support them, with information and advice.

Occupational therapists consider 'meaningful occupations' the things that a person wants, needs or chooses to do. This applies equally to the outdoor spaces adjacent to a person's home.

Do they have a vehicle and is this their main form of transport?

Who puts the bins out? How does the location for bin collection day relate to where the bins are stored the rest of the time?

Are they a keen gardener?

Is the garden a space for play and leisure?

So many questions!...

Adaptations and outside space should reflect the person's preferences and changing needs, including, but not exclusively linked to, their physical abilities. The emotional resonance of a space should be something that is considered whenever possible. Consider, for example:

- If a family pet is buried where you intend to create a parking area, this is something that the person will need to process. Is this a step too far? They may need time to consider the options.

- Does someone want to access a particular spot because that is where they always sat and relaxed with a family member who is no longer alive?

Although there may be other areas where access can be more easily achieved, do not automatically default to what is closest or cheapest, although this may be what can be facilitated. It is often the recognition of emotional ties that is more important than the end result.

Why do we need outside space?

Most people need and have connections to others. This may be stating the obvious; we have lived through lockdowns and realized that video calls are no replacement for face-to-face interactions – so supporting connectivity is essential. Leaving our homes serves many purposes, including health, wellbeing, education, leisure and play; it also provides us with connection to our communities, the area we live in and the people we interact with. This connection is practical, giving access to food, medicines, learning and work. However, communities comprise individuals and groups, and, given the choice and opportunity, we move between these to meet the requirements of the occupations we want or have to engage in. This engagement with our neighbourhood and community leads to a sense of belonging, contributing to a feeling of safety.

A lack of connection with others can be a contributing factor to mental health conditions, including anxiety and depression. Removing someone's access to their community is restrictive in many ways. In urban or semi-urban areas essential needs can be met via delivery services or online, but does this meet the human need for interactions with others? There will be some for whom this is a choice and preference. However, do not presume that where there are environmental barriers preventing access to the community that this situation is acceptable to the person you are supporting. This may seem obvious, but faced with the pressures of the role and limitations of funding and criteria, it is sometimes a position you may slip into. For occupational therapists this is actually an opportunity to proactively address health and other inequalities.

A dropped kerb and hardstanding do not just provide access to a vehicle, but are also opportunities for improved health, education, employment, and so many other opportunities!

The COVID-19 pandemic and lockdowns taught us the importance of outdoor space and its impact on health and wellbeing. Biophilia is the recognition that humans have a connection with nature, and gain health benefits from direct interaction with it. This is not to say that we should go out and hug trees on a regular basis, but we know that during lockdowns a lack of access to green space was cited by many as the most difficult aspect for people to manage.

Information-gathering

Occupational therapists are familiar with the concept of activity or task analysis. This highlights the barriers to an activity as well as the steps by which it is achieved. Taking the time to break down an activity can clarify what is necessary, appropriate and relevant to achieving intended outcomes, be that accessing a vehicle or hanging washing out. Follow the process through, to and from the dwelling or outdoor space, and consider how these spaces are linked. Is the occupation achieved? Can they do what you (or they) are aiming for?

Be realistic – how often do they hang the washing out? Would the most practical option be to relocate the washing line? But even before that, can they get the washing out of the machine, into a basket and out of the house? Breaking an activity down into its component parts identifies the areas of need, and assists professional reasoning in evidencing why you will (or will not) recommend a particular adaptation.

So far we have given you some rationale as to why removing barriers to access outside space is important. There needs to be guidance on what should be considered and how it can be achieved to back this up. As we have said, outside spaces come in many different forms, and we cannot provide definitive answers, but we have tried to cover most situations you will encounter.

Front and centre, making an entrance

Every property has some form of entrance, which is not always at the front, and not always visible as you approach the property. The entrance commonly used by visitors may not be the one that is most visible as you approach. Understanding how spaces are used and houses accessed is a part of information-gathering.

Pre-visit research

The internet provides a wealth of information and opportunity. Maps, street and satellite views, specific location identifiers, planning applications and property listings all provide information and valuable insight as to what to expect on a first visit. Online images will help you understand how a property is situated on its plot, access points and parking, and to identify any barriers or enablers. Any local knowledge supports this, as it is not always possible to see how steep a gradient is or how busy traffic is. Add to this a look at other properties in the area. Are there dropped kerbs and off-road parking? It is reasonable to expect this can be achieved if an identified need as a precedent has already been established.

Situation normal?

Most houses have direct access from some form of road, but not all. There are communal parking areas, green spaces with pathways... Shared access is more common than you may think. You may associate this with older properties away from main roads, but new developments have cul-de-sacs ending with a number of properties sharing communal access leading to individual drives and/or parking bays. This requires thought if you aim to provide access to the pavement and when recommending an adaptation that requires a significant build time, or large machinery that may impede neighbours' access.

First things first, let's look at the roadside:

- Is it a corner plot?

- Is a dropped kerb in place?

- Are there bus lanes, bus stops or restricted or resident parking?

- Any street furniture – lamp posts, post boxes, telegraph poles...?

- Are there trees or landscaping to consider?

- If there are shops, schools or other amenities, this may affect access, as will the type of road, nearby junctions or crossing points.

Some barriers will be such that you cannot resolve them. A pedestrian crossing where you want a dropped kerb and driveway? A corner plot on a junction with traffic lights? These are not things that can be changed, so your role may be to manage expectations. You can do many things, but miracles are not within your remit.

On-street parking

In an ideal world we would all be able to park outside our properties. This isn't always possible, and requests can be made for a dedicated accessible parking bay. In theory these should work well, but a note of caution. They cannot be designated for a single property or person (dependent on the area); while the bay may be provided, use by others may mean its provision makes no difference to the person it was intended to assist. This also applies with communal parking areas – anyone with a Blue Badge can use these bays. This is not saying to discount this option, but landlords and the Highways Department may be reluctant to consider it.

Off-road parking

First, a vehicle must be able to fit in the space available – it cannot block the pavement. Second, a dropped kerb is needed – this in itself takes some negotiation and coordination. The Highways Department has to give permission, and there are costs to consider. Then you need to know who owns the land between the kerb and the edge of the property. Don't presume there is an automatic right to drive a vehicle across this, and if there is an area of grass, this will need to be tarmacked. Your third consideration is the transition from the pavement to the front garden. Wall, fence or open plan? If there is a wall or a fence, who owns it? For rented properties, the landlord will need to give permission, or for shared or common areas neighbours (or their landlords) must give permission.

All this, and you haven't got into the front garden yet!

The final hurdle – the space in front of the property: is the front garden large enough for the type of vehicle used? This isn't as simple as the dimensions of the vehicle. You need to consider how the vehicle is accessed, as wheelchair-adapted vehicles may have side or rear access. Do the doors slide or swing open? Is there sufficient space for a wheelchair user to transfer out and then close the vehicle door?

Added to this, how else is the area used? Rubbish bins may be stored or wheeled across the area. Is there ramped access to the entrance?

Some other adjustments may be needed if you are to achieve the goal of off-road parking.

Many houses have garages, which are often used as storage areas, but don't assume this is the case. (Usually these properties will have access from the road, so that's part of the job already done.) Access to a garage may need to be maintained, so consider how a space is used. There's no point in creating a parking area for one vehicle to find its pattern of use prevents another being used.

Properties with shared spaces can be more complicated. There may be dedicated spaces allotted to a property or flat. If these are inaccessible due to the type of vehicle or needs of the person, what can be done? You should certainly be asking the relevant questions, as the outcome will depend on discussion or negotiation. Shared spaces with communal parking have similar issues to on-street parking and parking bays – they are dependent on others using the area. It is always worth approaching those with responsibility for the area – if you don't ask, you definitely won't get in this circumstance.

> Planning permission for off-road parking may be required. Our advice is to take advice, especially if it's a conservation area. Checking what is needed is easier than applying retrospectively. It isn't necessarily your role to determine if a planning application is needed; however, asking the question means that this can be considered.

Pathways

It makes sense that there will be access from the house to the pavement, but don't presume this is essential. (This may sound odd given the previous emphasis on access to the community.) You will have to balance need, necessity and planned use. Pathways to parking areas make sense, but beyond this, is a pathway needed? A pathway to the roadside when it is unlikely that it will be used to access a community or amenities is not an appropriate recommendation. Consider isolated rural locations on roads without pavements. How realistic is a path in this situation? Ensuring access to a vehicle, yes, but a pathway providing access to nowhere? Maybe not.

Pathways don't just lead away from properties – they also provide access to gardens and outside space – but their purpose must be identified. Is it to access a washing line, seating area or something else? Gardens come in many sizes and access to the whole area cannot be guaranteed. The DFG criteria specify access to the garden, but not the whole area. On a technicality the criteria could probably mean creating level access from the house, but more commonly this includes a small level area (or patio). Managing expectations can be difficult if the hope is that full access will be achieved through statutory funding. Where non-statutory funding is available, we can offer advice and guidance on the detail of the proposed schemes.

What should a pathway offer, and how does this differ from a ramp? Our interpretation is that a pathway uses existing topography (flat or sloped), while ramps address issues with topography. Building Regulations identify a pathway gradient of 1:60 as suitable (HM Government 2016). Part M of the Building Regulations (HM Government 2016) offers more guidance on pathways: Section 3 relates to access for wheelchair users, and Section 3.45 (p.50) advises that pathways should be a minimum width of 1050mm to private refuse, recycling or storage areas, and access to other areas 1500mm, with a minimum of 1500mm as a turning circle clear of obstruction.

While this is useful, it should be considered a starting point. You may be supporting someone with a wider than standard wheelchair, a person with a wide stance, or someone who walks with assistance and who needs a wider path. Turning areas must reflect the ability of the wheelchair user or attendant. Some may be able to turn on a sixpence, but others may be limited by upper limb strength, reach or stamina, and require a larger area. Consider needs beyond mobility – those with visual impairments may require highlighted edges and start and finish points, which could be via colour or the use of tactile paving, and supported by lighting.

Surface finishes

Part M of the Building Regulations (HM Government 2016) advises that a suitable ground surface is required, but what does this actually mean? It is easier to say what isn't appropriate. Loose surface options should be avoided. Finishes such as gravel and bark do not provide a usable surface, for either wheelchair or ambulant users. To this list you can add cobbles, crazy paving or anything similar.

Aesthetics play a part in the choice of surface finish. Concrete for a hardstanding and pathway can meet assessed needs, but may not 'match' the property's aesthetics. In these instances you can request costs for alternative finishes, as sometimes block paving has a similar cost.

Additional considerations are upkeep and longevity. Poured surfaces (concrete, tarmac, resin) and exposed aggregate provide smooth surface finishes with minimal upkeep. Pavers, setts and slabs will require more maintenance, and over time may lift and need resetting. Tree roots close to any paved area may result in an uneven surface later, and weeds will exploit any weakness in a surface.

> While it may be tempting to fully cover the area in front of a property with a smooth, accessible surface, there are other considerations unrelated to accessibility. Kelly (2018) highlights the impact of rainwater run-off from domestic dwellings as a factor increasing flooding in the UK. Drainage channels can reduce the amount of run-off, and a designed soakaway and areas of planting or permeable or semipermeable surface finishes can also play a part.

Handrails and upstands
Depending on how a person mobilizes, you may not require handrails; however, if the pathway is more than 60mm above the adjacent ground level, handrails and upstands are required (for more details, see Chapter 18).

Lighting
This is something that should be considered alongside parking and pathways. Lighting provides a sense of security and safety as well as assisting with safe use. It is not something that is usually considered in isolation, with most properties having some form of external lighting. Your role is to consider if additional or new lighting is needed, and if you need to seek statutory funding for provision.

Could an identified need be met via solar lights? These are readily available and can be wall- or post-mounted and don't require a qualified electrician. Is lighting related to a recommendation for adaptation? This may serve a new access point or if an adaptation obscures an existing light. Will the light highlight a specific point, such as a lock, assisting someone to independently open their front door?

Lights can be inset in paths or steps, or within a handrail highlighting the ground, thereby reducing the risk of trips or falls.

Hidden hazards
For pathways and hardstandings much of the cost is taken up through ground preparation and foundations. The utilities serving a property may affect plans or increase costs. Although not immediately apparent, drains,

sewerage and power supplies for the property may run through the area. Noting the location of manhole covers and meter cupboards assists in planning.

Barriers and boundaries

Barriers aren't always a negative thing, as fences and gates, for example, define the curtilage or extent of a property. For some, barriers are essential to promote safety (see Chapter 17). Fences are not usually barriers to access, but the type of gate and latch used will affect accessibility.

Gates

Removing a gate will promote access, but this is not always the preferred option; depending on an area, gates may promote security, and reduce anxiety associated with personal safety.

The weight of the gate itself should be considered and the force required to open and close it. Part M of the Building Regulations advises that the force to open a domestic door should not exceed 20 Newtons (HM Government 2016), so it is not unreasonable to consider this as appropriate for gates. As you probably won't have access to equipment to measure Newtons, what is more relevant is to assess if the person using that access point can use the gate. Alongside this, any latch or handle will need to be at a usable height and of a suitable design.

Just remember that a gate is only as good as its use. If it is not secured by those using it, it will not be effective. And it's not just family members – visitors and post and delivery drivers may not appreciate the need to secure a gate.

Fences

Generally fencing is considered the property owner's responsibility, but where the person's safety is an identified need, there are some options to consider. Where low-level fences are already installed and there are safety concerns, standard fence panels are unlikely to be funded by a DFG, but a social housing landlord may consider provision.

If 'standard' fencing panels need to be changed, you may need advice. If the issue is linked to the person absconding or climbing the fence, the difference between horizontal or vertical slats may be all that is needed. Horizontal designs support climbing more than vertical slats. Also consider the orientation of the fence panels if they are braced by horizontal backer rails, which traditionally face into the owner's garden; this may need discussion and negotiation with neighbours. If a neighbour's fence panels are installed with the framework facing into the garden you need to secure, you could add an additional fence inside the boundary to provide the required smooth surface finish. Composite fence panels provide a smooth finish that doesn't offer grip or foot holds, making them more difficult to scale.

Standard fencing may not resolve the issue, especially if the person is determined to leave the property or enjoys the sensation of climbing but has no sense of safety or risk. Here, specialist or non-standard provision alternatives may be required and are more likely to be considered for statutory funding. These include anti-scale fencing or roller barriers that are set above the standard fence height, or even anti-climb coating.[1]

Don't forget the view the household will see daily – if the outdoor space looks like an industrial site or prison, it reduces the likelihood it will be used. Potentially efforts may be made to obscure the fence, defeating its purpose, as these will provide opportunities to climb. For more information on managing safety, use this information in conjunction with Chapter 17.

Gardens

Access to outdoor space is important for both health and wellbeing. Depending on your role and remit, while access to and use of a garden space may not be considered a priority, before moving on, think about what you know about the person you are supporting. Your information-gathering and conversations will have provided transferable information. If they have fatigue or pain, the suggestion of rest points is appropriate. For those who are unsteady when mobilizing, handrails along pathways or adjacent to steps promote safety. Where reach or balance is compromised, installation of raised beds may be the solution. And so on...

These are not recommendations that require you to identify sources of funding, just advice that can be offered if it is felt appropriate. If circumstances allow, you can make recommendations, utilize existing knowledge, apply activity/task analysis and the PEOP (Person-Environment-Occupation-Performance) model to enable and support access. You don't need to be a horticulturist or gardener, however, as your role is to promote access, not create a planting scheme.

---

1   www.insight-security.com/roller-barrier-non-aggressive-anti-climb-spinners

Not all adaptations will relate to permanent changes. Sensory gardens can enable someone with dementia to recall memories through scent, or a scent pathway can guide someone who is visually impaired. The need for vestibular stimulation for those with sensory-processing disorders may mean access to a trampoline, swing or slide. You may not be responsible for providing these, but facilitating access may fall within your remit.

Storage

There are two types of storage to consider: for vehicles and for leisure. If the property has a garage, a vehicle may be stored in it when not in use; it is, however, highly unlikely that statutory funding will provide for a garage space to be built. If a vehicle is always garaged and is driven by the person you are supporting, assessing transfers in and out of their vehicle in this space is reasonable, as is advice on door opening systems. If the vehicle is electric, access to a charge point will also need to be considered.

Do not presume that the vehicle the person uses is a car or a van; their transport may be a bicycle, adapted trike or powered wheelchair, and mobility scooters and powered wheelchairs also need to be stored and charged. In most instances responsibility for overnight storage will lie with the owner of the scooter or wheelchair. Landlords may specify the location or type of storage, and covenants or restrictions may apply that influence options. As an occupational therapist these issues are not for you to resolve, but knowing about this should be helpful in managing expectations.

Storage for leisure activities isn't something that usually falls within an occupational therapist's remit. Then again, if a shed is inaccessible or at a distance, suggesting that it or an alternative is located closer to the dwelling isn't unreasonable, even though you won't be in a position to facilitate this.

Other barriers and enablers: red tape

These are not the physical barriers mentioned previously. You may, for instance, find that an enquiry is met with a response that indicates that there is a 'blanket policy' in place:

'We never do fences.'

'Access to the garden isn't considered essential.'

'Driveways or off-road parking is only for full-time wheelchair users.'

The relevant adaptation policy for the organization is your friend – even if it specifies that they do not provide something you have identified as a need. In the RCOT Specialist Section – Housing briefing paper *Home Adaptations, the Care Act 2014 and related provision across the UK* (RCOT 2016), Michael Mandelstam advises that 'housing authorities need to be aware of government guidance about the 2002 Order warning against blanket policies not to provide assistance – in order to avoid an unlawful fettering of discretion', this references the 2003 Housing Renewal Circular from the Office of the Deputy Prime Minister[2] (ODPM 2003).

An organization's adaptation policies will provide you with the parameters for decision-making that they have applied. These will facilitate discussions when a request is denied. Your identification of a need that is based on completion of an assessment will enable you to challenge any 'blanket policy' as you will be able to provide your professional reasoning as to why the person's medical condition or diagnosis supports provision of an adaptation.

Other barriers include the unexpected Tree Preservation Order (TPO), the listing of a building, location in a conservation area or restrictive covenants. All except covenants can be identified via the local council or authority website, usually in both list and map form. TPOs relate to specific trees; however, within conservation areas there are limits to works on all trees, and permission is required for trees of a certain size, even for pruning branches. Restrictive covenants are generally highlighted when a building is purchased, so owners are usually aware; if there is any doubt, details can be purchased from the Land Registry for the relevant country in the UK. These are not the remit of the person making recommendations, although it is useful to be aware of anything that might put a spanner in the works.

In this chapter we have tried to highlight the benefits of promoting and facilitating access to outdoor space. This may be as a way of accessing the opportunities in the wider community or a leisure area. There are some challenges when making recommendations to make outdoor spaces accessible, but these should not put you off from trying to address them. Hopefully the information here has prepared you to assess the space available, identify appropriate needs and solutions, and to complete a recommendation that is supported by your professional reasoning.

---

2   Now the Department for Levelling Up, Housing and Community (DLUHC).

20

Kitchen Adaptations

Knowledge check

* What can you learn from a hot drink assessment?

* List 12 aspects of your observation that will inform your decision-making in regard to the kitchen environment.

* Think about physical, cognitive and emotional aspects that you will be able to identify from an assessment.

How we use our kitchen varies, but we all complete activities to prepare food and drink. The available space, for example, dictates its use. Narrow galley kitchens aren't conducive to family gatherings, and make it difficult for two people to work at the same time. Larger rooms or open-plan layouts mean that kitchens can be social spaces, becoming multi-purpose areas supporting socialization, work, education and leisure.

So how do we unpick this? Start, as always, with the person. Your assessment will allow you to understand how they use the space within their home, as well as how they manage tasks and activities.

Mealtimes span the whole day, and we need drinks to prevent dehydration, but it goes beyond this. Preparation of food and drink may be a key part of a person's role within their household, culturally, arising from a specific interest or from family routines. Routines around food and drink extend to guests and visitors. How often do we welcome guests by asking if they want or need something to eat or drink? Retaining independence in this area supports these societal norms and customs, enabling people to continue with their preferred routines.

Meals vary widely, from solitary meals for one, to large social gatherings, meals prepared from fresh ingredients, to ready meals that just need reheating. Once we understand how often and the way a space is used we can look more closely at the way activities are completed. An activity or task analysis can be used to consider the complex mix between person, occupation and environment. This occupational therapy tool will enable you to consider all the elements of an activity or occupation, and to identify where support or an adaptation is required.

In kitchens you will need to understand the physical abilities required to complete what can appear to be 'simple, everyday' tasks. Standing balance, mobility, range of movement, grip and stamina are a few physical requirements to consider. Then you need to consider the cognitive aspects of activities – sequencing, concentration and memory all play a part.

Much of this can be gathered without observing specific tasks; you will see the person moving around their home, observing aspects such as grip as they open doors, noting stamina or shortness of breath. Conversations and discussions will have highlighted some cognitive issues such as recall. And, of course, there is always the opportunity to observe them making you a drink if they (a) offer you one and (b) you want one!

Consider the ubiquitous hot drink assessment so often used in occupational therapy. This is a familiar activity providing a significant amount of information. This includes (although this is not an exhaustive list) the following:

Physical	Cognitive	Emotional
Gait	Initiate the task	**Presentation**
Balance	Recall	**Affect**
Range of movement	Memory (long and short term)	**Mood**
Reach	Sequencing	**Motivation**
Fine/gross motor skills	Concentration	**Anxiety**
Patterns of movement	Orientation in time	
Stamina	Processing auditory and visual information	
Grip	Problem-solving	
Tremor	Safety	
Eye-hand coordination	Object identification	
Vision		

Does this match the list you created from the knowledge check at the beginning of the chapter?

This list applies to any task in the kitchen, but you won't have time to observe each and every task, from preparing drinks and meals to doing the laundry. Your observations will enable you to identify any barriers, and from this, to identify possible solutions. Remember that the solutions don't always have to be high-tech; sometimes, simple changes such as altering where items are stored or adding labels is sufficient.

Having identified any barriers, you need to consider what you can recommend to promote independence and safety. Kitchen layouts reflect the space available, and you will often need to work with what you are given. Kitchen designers recommend that the key items of sink, hob and refrigerator are located in a triangle, referred to as the 'golden triangle', as this is the most ergonomic layout.

The most common kitchen layouts are:

- *Galley kitchens*, which are long and usually narrow, with units on one or both sides. Often there is only enough space between the cabinets for one person to work, limiting options for assistance or for use of a wheelchair, mobility aid or perching stool. Galley kitchens may not be spacious, but their design requires people to move between cupboards more frequently, increasing effort. Access to items stored in base units or to the oven may be hampered by lack of space to bend and reach. On the plus side there is a limited distance between work surfaces, enabling the transfer of items between work surface, sink and hob.

- *U-shaped kitchens*, which are considered to be the most accessible design, meeting the needs of a wide range of users. They allow for installation of the three key items in a triangle, but, if space between units is limited, and similar to galley kitchens, they may lack space for those with physical limitations. For wheelchair users, installation of higher than standard kickboards may provide some additional room for manoeuvring.

- *L-shaped kitchens*, which have two open sides, providing additional floor space and promoting access for many users, and can allow for seating to be situated in the kitchen. This design still allows for the configuration of hob, sink and refrigerator in a triangle.

- *Open-plan kitchens*, which are likely to follow the designs above, but without a door to consider when accessing them. This is a positive if space between units allows for easy access when island units are included.

- *Utility rooms* have become commonplace in modern house design. While not a kitchen, they do house items that relate to kitchen tasks, including fridges, freezers, microwaves, washing machines and tumble dryers. It may be that relocating some white goods from a utility room into the kitchen is required to promote independence.

Food and drink preparation requires a suitable work surface or kitchen table. Kitchen work surfaces are generally installed to enable food preparation when the person is standing, which makes it difficult for those who prefer or need to sit down. The simplest option is to use a table and chair, but if there is insufficient space, you can create an area by removing a base unit (or two) and lowering a section of work surface. The height of this will need to allow for the person's thighs when seated, allowing for clearance as they wheel into position (if they use a wheelchair).

The need to be specific on work surface height can be negated through installing a height-adjustable work surface. These can be manually operated or powered, so consider who will be operating it and setting the height. For shared spaces, or for a person who prefers to stand for some activities, this enables changes in height without relocating ingredients or kitchen utensils etc. This option reduces base unit storage space, which may be an issue in smaller spaces where the person cannot reach the wall units. An alternative to a lowered work surface is a pull-out or fold-down one that can be stored away when not required. Similarly, a pull-out ironing board can be installed, enabling access and use.

To support transfer of items to and from the hob or sink, kitchen designs should incorporate a work surface on either side of the hob or sink, with heat-resistant surfaces supporting those who cannot lift hot or heavy items. Heat protection strips or 'hot rods' can be applied to the work surface, although these prevent items being slid across and could cause pans to tip. (It's also worth considering how work surfaces are joined – metal joining strips create a raised area.)

Sinks

The choice of sink designs available today is huge, and taps no longer simply dispense hot and cold water, adding to decision-making. Aesthetics come into play, and an advantage of an abundance of choice is that it should be possible to find something that is both in keeping with a person's taste and is functional and usable.

A sink should not be too deep, especially if the person using it will be seated. If possible, avoid circular designs, as it is easier to locate items in a rectangular bowl than a round one. Ceramic sinks are 'unforgiving' if crockery or glassware is dropped or placed heavily. The deep, ceramic butler sink is possibly not the 'go to' choice of sink. The traditional stainless steel sink design has lasted simply because it functions well. Fear not, though – there are contenders. Resin sinks are available in a range of colours and styles, and it should be possible to identify something suitable.

It is possible to install a sink in a rise and fall unit as long as the correct fittings are used and the hoses do not intrude into the open area as they may get entangled, and as the person moves away, become disconnected.

Finally, lifting a full washing-up bowl requires grip and strength, so a wire basket may be appropriate.

Do you choose the sink or the tap(s) first? The sink dictates the type of tap as it has either one or two holes. So do you assess the tap design first? A conundrum...

Taps

As tap design and function has evolved, it is now possible to have a tap supplying hot, cold, filtered, sparkling and boiling water. Even with all these choices you still need to consider its position (can it be reached?) and the method of operation. Lever or turn-handle designs are traditional, but sensor taps are available. First and foremost, though, having a design where hot and cold feeds are easily identified is vital.

On the selection of taps, monobloc taps may have a single lever or handle, which, depending on design, may not be as easy to use as two taps or bridge units. When specifying lever taps in a scheme, be sure to include the length of the lever as some designs are minimalist and may be difficult for someone with a reduced range of movement. A monobloc tap with a high swivel spout makes filling pots and kettles easier as they can be placed on the work surface rather than held over the sink.

Finally, boiling water taps: these remove the need to lift a kettle (and waiting for it to boil). However, any tap with a filter system will need this to be changed, so who completes that task must be considered. (Activity analysis identifies that if the filter is installed in a base unit, the lucky person will need to be flexible, with good eye–hand coordination as well as a strong grip.)

Storage

Good storage solutions make kitchen space more useable. Consider a person's reach, which may be restricted by musculoskeletal conditions such as osteoarthritis affecting their shoulder joint. A person's working position impacts reach. This may result from scoliosis or kyphosis limiting spinal extension, or from the need to work in a seated position.

Base units can provide suitable storage, but items at the rear of cupboards may still be inaccessible. Pull-out baskets or shelves on runners resolve this issue, as do the use of drawer units. Base units don't always have to be floor-based; it may be that by mounting them slightly higher they are more accessible for wheelchair users.

Wall units are more of a challenge as they are inaccessible to most wheelchair users and the highest shelves inaccessible for many. It may be that these aren't used if there is sufficient storage in base units, but what if there is limited space available? Pull-down units can be fitted into cupboards with manual or powered operation, reducing the effort required. Cupboards can be set on vertical runners with a powered mechanism, and lowered as and when required.

Open shelves offer clarity and ease of access as long as they are within reach. Without the need to open doors, items placed on shelves are accessible and potentially more easily located. Freestanding cupboards provide flexibility in where they are located. Larder cupboards are often shallower, and utilize the doors as storage space, making the contents more visible and accessible.

Cupboard doors and handles also play their part:

- Glazed doors increase visibility.

- Doors hinged to open upwards may be out of reach for those with a limited range of movement.

- Bar-type handles are more easily gripped than small knobs.

- A strong contrast between cupboard door finishes and handles assists those who have a visual impairment.

White goods

White goods (and gadgets) are part of every kitchen. Fridges and freezers can be freestanding or under-counter, individual units or combined, cupboard-style, countertop or drawer units – whatever works in the space and for the person you are working with. Dishwashers with pull-out drawers are usually accessible, ideally located so they can be accessed from both sides rather than adjacent to a wall.

Low-profile electric hobs allow for transfer of pans more easily, but may have touch controls that are harder to locate. Designs vary in the number of rings for cooking, with some 'zoned' rather than having defined rings, allowing for different shapes of pans. They also have an indicator light to indicate that there is residual heat on the hob. Gas hobs have more controllable heat levels, but pans cannot be slid to one side as easily. Although it is often best to continue with the hob type that someone is familiar with, it is still worth a discussion.

Hobs can be installed at a height to suit wheelchair users or those who need to sit while cooking, and on height-adjustable surfaces. What needs consideration, though, is heat transfer below the hob on to the person's thighs, high temperatures or prolonged exposure to heat.

The position of the grill depends on what type of oven is fitted. If possible, avoid eye-level grills above hobs. Built-in ovens can be installed below the hob or in tower units. These units offer options for the height of the oven and grill, so their positioning can reflect the needs of the person. Drop-down doors provide a (hot) surface to place dishes on as they are moved in and out of the oven, and, like dishwashers, ovens are better placed with access from both sides. If space is at a premium there are ovens with doors that slide into a recess under the oven, but this usually reduces the oven capacity.

Agas, Rayburns and similar range-style ovens can provide constant heat and options for cooking, but the weight of the doors and hob covers may be an issue, as is the reach required to lift the hob cover. Microwave ovens can be countertop or installed within units. They offer flexibility, and, depending on the design, may offer more than one cooking method. They can be repositioned on countertops, and may remove the need to use the oven.

It goes without saying that smoke or heat and carbon monoxide detectors should be installed (and tested), but it is always worth repeating. The Fire and Rescue Service usually has a safety check service, providing and installing detectors for vulnerable people and their families.

There are numerous other gadgets designed to make our lives easier but that can end up cluttering up work surfaces and reducing workspace.

Air fryers are safer than chip pans; toasters have a lower fire risk than using the grill; hot water dispensers and coffee machines reduce the need to lift heavy kettles... When suggesting that countertops are cleared, make recommendations based on what is used rather than focusing on the size of the gadget and the space to be gained. You don't want to create space to work but raise the risk of an injury.

Finally in this section are extraction units – not technically a gadget or white goods, but essential, especially if the person cannot easily open a window. Extractor hoods above the hob may be difficult to reach, but alternative designs are available that retract into the worktop or that are operated via remote control.

Power sockets and lighting

Gadgets need power and good lighting supports safety, so both need to be planned into any adaptation. First, power sockets – in our opinion, you can never have enough! The aim is to avoid trailing leads and to locate sockets where they are needed. Installing pull-up sockets provides flexibility and can reduce the need to reach across work surfaces to operate them.

Kitchens are lit by natural light, but this is dependent on the window size, orientation, weather conditions and how clean the glazing is. Ensuring that the whole kitchen is well lit supports safe use, but additional lighting in task-specific locations is recommended. This could be via ceiling-mounted spot or downlighters, lighting installed under wall cupboards or ensuring the cooker hood has an integral light.

Rubbish

Waste disposal has become complicated, with different rules, regulations and a bewildering array of wheelie bins, so you can't be too specific in your recommendations. Councils have arrangements in place for those who cannot manage to take out their wheelie bin. The need to sort out different types of waste (landfill, recycling, paper, food...) may mean that there are three or more bins that can end up cluttering up the kitchen area. Consider bins with internal dividers, reducing the number of bins. If there is sufficient storage space, pull-out designs can be installed in base units, but these are then hidden from view and may make identification difficult.

The complexity of activities that take place in the kitchen means that this chapter can only skim the surface of what should be considered. Promoting independence and ease of access supports much more than meeting nutritional needs, although health benefits from a good diet cannot be understated. The ability to complete kitchen-based tasks reduces dependence on others, promoting autonomy and choice.

21

Toilet Adaptations

Toileting is not an activity that is often discussed openly. Independence in toileting is a key milestone for toddlers, and a frequent discussion point for parents of young children. Not all children achieve this within the expected age range – some are developmentally delayed and others will not become continent. For adults it is commonly expected that they will be continent and able to manage their own intimate cleanliness after using the toilet.

As an occupational therapist you will come in as a stranger, expecting those you are working with to be open with you, whereas their instinct is most likely to avoid what can be considered a private or taboo subject. This may be due to a cultural influence or simply embarrassment – and you may be feeling the same as well. The potential for misunderstanding is significant!

Place yourself in the metaphorical shoes of a 16-year-old teenager sitting with a parent and being asked to describe exactly how they manage to clean themselves after opening their bowels, if they stand to urinate or how they manage menstruation. Next, imagine you are in your 80s needing a son, daughter or caregiver to support you, having to ask when you need to go to the toilet. While it is unlikely you would be comfortable with either scenario, this is the reality for many of those you work with.

You need and must ask the awkward questions to fully understand one of the most private occupations we have. Understanding how the person uses the toilet takes in routine, culture, preference, cognition and physical ability. Just because you sit on a toilet with your back to the cistern doesn't mean that the person you are working with does as well. Cleansing after using the toilet may mean using paper or wet wipes. What if they wash using a bidet or shower attachment? More to consider...

Once you fully understand the way a person manages toileting, you then need to understand what (if any) changes they are able to accept. Cultural or religious beliefs may mean that they want to retain the same practice or method.

There may be medical reasons that mean changes to enable access to a toilet are needed, including restricted mobility or fatigue. Changes to bladder and bowel control may result in frequency or urgency, or the opposite, bowel movements taking longer – which is potentially an issue in households with a single toilet. Other reasons to consider access to a toilet include self-catheterization, bowel irrigation, enemas or stoma care. None of these require a toilet for sole use by one person, but a holistic assessment will identify if there is an impact on toilet availability for the person or for those they live with.

Children may have a delay in becoming aware of the need to urinate or open their bowels, and parents may request installation of an additional toilet to support a toileting programme. This will need some consideration, as it is not possible to provide a toilet simply to initiate a programme where it is hoped that a child might become continent. You will need evidence that they have shown some awareness, that there is professional support for the programme, and that there will be support across other settings to provide consistency to ensure that the toileting programme will be effective. A pragmatic approach is to wait until there is evidence of progress in another setting (usually educational).

A note on commodes: These are effective short-term solutions for toileting needs, and may be appropriate for use overnight for the less mobile. As they need emptying, this may mean that independence is not achieved if a person is unable to empty the commode pan themselves. It may be that a toilet adaptation reduces the need for caregiver support, which not only promotes privacy and dignity, but also contributes to reduction of pressure on social care resources.

Now let's consider some practicalities of toilet adaptations.

Location

Domestic dwellings typically have toilets on the same floor as the bedrooms, but some older properties such as terraced houses may have toilets (and bathrooms) on the ground floor, often adjacent to the kitchen. Either way, in properties with more than one storey and toilet facilities on a single floor, there is always a period in the day where a person needs to climb or descend stairs to access the toilet.

Adding an additional toilet is not always the answer. If a person has reduced mobility and stairs are a challenge, then other rooms are less accessible, so a stairlift or through floor lift will promote access to toilet facilities alongside other rooms.

Toilet design

Toilets come in all shapes and sizes, some more practical than others. If seat height is an issue, don't immediately think 'let's add a plinth' or a different design. The humble raised toilet seat (RTS) is a low-tech option that should always be your initial solution. This may not work for all, such as those who complete sideways transfers, but don't dismiss the RTS out of hand.

The bog standard (sorry, we couldn't let the opportunity pass!) design of toilets works well for most. Usually, they are compatible with most equipment (RTS, frame, combined toilet seat and frame etc.) and forgiving to those whose ability to lower themselves down to sit is reduced. Wall-hung toilets with concealed cisterns look smart and suit modern bathroom design, but can prevent commodes from being positioned directly over the bowl. Without the support of a pedestal they may not support obese people or those who sit down heavily. Bowl design presents similar problems, as the bowl may be too short to match a commode aperture, especially for those who sit sacrally.

Flush handles and type

Most toilets have side-mounted lever flush handles or push-button controls, top- or side-mounted. Lever flush handles can be operated in a number of ways – with a flat hand, fist or even an elbow. Larger paddle types or longer levers make operation easier.

Push-button flushes require more eye–hand coordination and may be difficult for someone with a tremor. The force required to push down is directed through just one or two fingers, which, for those with an arthritic condition, may be painful to use, and for some require excessive downward force.

High-level cisterns with pull chains are a traditional style that is still available today, and may be installed to reflect the aesthetic properties of older properties. They share one of the challenges presented by push-button operations, however, in that good eye–hand coordination and motor control is needed to grasp the pull chain.

Bidet seat or wash and dry toilet?

Wash and dry toilets have been viewed as either something only experienced when on holiday in Japan, or solely as an adaptation for disabled people. This is no longer the case, although increased availability and mainstream provision does not necessarily make things easier.

There are several wash and dry toileting options. The first is a bidet seat; this has the same functionality as a wash and dry toilet, but is designed to replace just the standard toilet seat. However, it requires a suitable power and water supply and usually has fewer settings, which may mean it cannot be programmed to meet the person's specific needs.

Wash and dry toilets can be purchased from a number of bathroom suppliers and may meet need. Where you will need to investigate further is the options for user controls, settings for the wash arm and compatibility with toileting or shower chairs. If a toileting or shower chair is, or is likely, to be needed, there are models that are compatible with wash and dry toilets (usually Geberit or Closomat, but the market continues to expand). You will need to assess both the type of toilet chair and the model of toilet, and find the most appropriate combination.

An en suite or family bathroom?

There can be a presumption that meeting assessed need must be via an en-suite facility. This is not the case, especially if it reduces available space. If the family bathroom can be adapted, this often provides more space than an en suite, allowing for repositioning of a toilet to maximize transfer options. On the other hand, it may be that swapping a person's bedroom to the master bedroom with an en suite is what is needed – although this is not always an option that is welcomed!

Toilet position

Toilets are traditionally placed close to walls, which is great for fitting grab rails, but less so if it prevents provision of equipment, or if the transfer method requires access from that side, or if transferring on one side and off the other.

Toilets are connected to waste pipes, and ideally these should exit directly behind the toilet, but systems may be designed with the waste pipe running at 90°, often 'boxed in' to hide pipework. This configuration often affects the use of toilet chairs as it prevents them being positioned fully over the toilet bowl.

You will also need to consider caregivers who need space to offer support, and who may have their own physical limitations. There may just be one informal caregiver, or there may be a care package in place with a number of different caregivers throughout the day.

There's no single answer to this conundrum, just awareness that it is much like chess, with one move impacting on other activities. For example, moving the toilet can affect access to the basin or the bath. The challenge with toilets is that they are usually in a small room with other fixed items, and are reliant on both water supply and waste outlets.

Grab rails

We will keep this brief as rails are focused on in more detail in Chapter 18. Observation of toilet transfers highlights when the basin, radiator or towel rail is used to assist. None of these are designed to support the angled force applied during transfers, which means that, over time, they will become loose and may pose a risk. Appropriate rails installed in an optimal position will promote safe transfers that require less effort.

Tilt or full-rise toilet seats

There are toilet seats that tilt or assist to rise, and may be considered equipment rather than an adaptation, but they are an option to consider. These, like RTS or fixed-toilet supports, must have their installation assessed in regard to the needs of others in the household accessing the toilet. They may assist one person but then prevent others using the toilet, which, if this is the only toilet in the property, defeats their purpose.

Emergency access and door hinges

Toileting is usually carried out in private, which can raise concerns if a person is at risk of a fall, a seizure or becoming ill. If the space is limited and the toilet door opens inwards, it will make offering assistance more difficult.

The first thing to consider is the type of lock installed. If a lock is routinely used, then installing a design that can be opened from the outside in the event of an emergency is an initial step. Then consider the way the door opens. If it opens into the room, can it be altered to open outwards? What is the impact of this change on the area and fittings such as light switches? If it's not appropriate to change the way the door is opened, there are still options. Hinges can be changed to designs where the vertical pin can be removed and then the door lifted away. Alternatively hinges designed to move 180° allow the door to be opened inwards during everyday use and outwards in an emergency.

Separate bathrooms and toilets are often situated either side of a dividing wall. It may seem sensible to increase space by removing the wall, which is a frequent adaptation request, but first, take time to consider how this is going to impact the access of other family members if this is the only toilet facility in the house. If the person's self-care or bathing routine takes time to complete, this may prevent access to the toilet for other members of the household. We are not saying that you should discount this option, but do ensure that this has been discussed before bringing out the sledgehammer!

Occupational therapists spend a lot of time in toilets and bathrooms, as these are where the barriers to self-care occupations are most frequently found. This chapter can be considered on its own or alongside Chapter 22, reflecting the situation you are assessing. There are rarely straightforward answers, but we offer a few options to consider, and from these you can develop additional ones as your level of experience grows.

22

Bathroom Adaptations

Knowledge check

* What is the difference between a basin and a sink?

* What is the difference between a wet room and a level-access shower?

We have separated bathroom and toilet adaptations into two chapters, as, although they are often required within the same room, they support very different activities. Therefore, this chapter focuses on bathing and showering.

Like toileting, bathing is usually completed in privacy, but generally speaking, a conversation and discussion about how this is achieved causes less embarrassment. There is still a need to have a full discussion, however, as how we achieve personal cleanliness will differ. Some people will be flexible and not mind if they have a bath or a shower, whereas others will be clear in what they want or need. The choice between bathing and showering is not just personal preference, but linked to sensory processing, culture, belief, and for some, a medical need.

Your assessment will identify bathing methods, barriers, enablers and preferences, and these should be considered alongside your evaluation of the bathroom environment – size, layout and facilities.

In most instances a decision will need to be made between bathing and showering. If the adaptation is funded via a DFG, the wording in the legislation supports access to both bathing and showering; however, a pragmatic approach is required. There may not be the space to achieve this, and the costs of achieving it may exceed the available funds. If both can be achieved and your assessment indicates they are both needed, it is appropriate that your recommendation reflects this.

Understanding a person's physical and cognitive abilities will guide your decision-making. If they are unable to safely step into a bath, consider equipment first before recommending installation of a shower. If they are able to lift their legs over into a bath when seated, then a bath lift is probably your first option. We suggest, based on experience and professional reasoning, that the 'belt-type' bath lifts are, for most, not appropriate. They do not offer a firm base of support and lack a back rest for those who need trunk support. Bath lifts offer these but need to be lifted in and out from the base of the bath, which may be a barrier for others in the household – both for bathing and for cleaning the bath.

Another consideration is caregiver support. Does the room offer sufficient space for a caregiver? Does the caregiver have any physical limitations that may affect how they can offer support to someone sitting in the bath? Consider their need to kneel, bend and reach when supporting bathing.

There may be a medical reason for bathing rather than showering, such as for skin conditions. If emollients are used, these can leave an oily film on the bath surface, which increases the risk of slips during transfers. A slip-resistant bathmat is always recommended, but the addition of well-placed grab rails will also assist, with advice to ensure hands are dried before use.

There can be a preconception that for those with a diagnosis of epilepsy or a history of seizures bathing is not appropriate. This is not the case, and any decision must be evidence-based. What is the seizure pattern? How well controlled is their epilepsy? What type of seizure do they experience, and do they have any pre-seizure symptoms? If there is evidence that they can continue to bathe safely and this is their preference, and they have capacity to make this decision, you should look to support positive risk-taking.

Sensory preferences will direct choice. If a person cannot tolerate a bathing method, this can cause discomfort or distress. Therefore, a change from a bath to a shower (or vice versa) should be supported, if it has been evidenced that the alternative is appropriate.

Location

Where should a bathroom be? Is an en suite essential for those with disabilities? If a family bathroom can be effectively adapted and is appropriate, then no. It is situational and reflects the house layout, the assessed needs and practicality. If an en suite is created and the person needs hoisting between this and the bedroom, consider a design where the dividing wall is lower and no dividing door fitted. This often allows for full coverage of the space, with a tracked hoist offering increased flexibility and usability.

Lighting

Effective lighting will increase safety in what can be considered a high-risk area – the smooth surfaces of baths, showers and floors combined with water pose risks for many. For safety, bathroom lighting has to comply with BS 7671 (BSI 2018), and is zoned according to proximity to water or moisture. An internet search will provide links to sites that illustrate these zones.

Modern houses often have bathrooms in the centre of the property with no natural light, making the choice of artificial lighting key. Bathrooms are often filled with white gloss, chrome and mirrored surfaces, making glare an issue for some. Downlighters are often used in bathrooms and provide good coverage. One disadvantage is that for those who are in a reclined position, such as lying in the bath, in a tilt-in-space shower chair or on a changing or shower bench, the light emitted can be uncomfortable for them. If providing downlighters in a new scheme, avoid installing them directly above areas where this may be an issue.

How a room is lit includes the method of control. Light switches are used outside of the room and light pulls within the bathroom. For those with cognitive impairment a light switch may not appear connected to the operation of lighting in the bathroom. On the other hand, a light pull requires good eye–hand coordination and reach to operate. Light pulls are usually supplied with a white cord, which may not be visible. For task lighting, such as at the basin, sensor lighting requires less control to operate and can be integrated into a mirror or bathroom cabinet.

Access

The bathroom is often the smallest room in the house, with the narrowest door. The typical position on the landing adjacent to bedrooms and the limited space in the room may mean that this is challenging to resolve. Removing the doorstop may provide a little additional width, but consider equipment options including the use of a ceiling track hoist for those who are not mobile. Another option is to consider if a second or different access to the room can be created, but this, in part, will depend on the room layout, adjacent rooms and the needs of others in the household. It may be that the room must be made larger or an additional bathroom facility (en suite) has to be created, but this may affect the size and number of bedrooms available.

Sink or basin

First, is it a sink or a basin? What's the difference? In reality, very little. Basins are smaller and situated in bathrooms (and may be called a bathroom sink!); both have taps and wastes with a stopper. Here we use 'basin' to differentiate between the wash facility in a bathroom and that in a kitchen ('sink').

Wash hand basin design offers a wide range of choice and style, with wall-hung, semi-pedestal, pedestal and countertop most common, although there are toilet designs with basins integrated into the top of the cistern where space is limited. Pedestal designs have greater stability than wall-hung basins, and may be more appropriate for someone who leans on it during use (but not using the basin as a transfer aid!). Wall-hung basins allow access for wheelchair users and those who need to sit while washing their hands or cleaning their teeth. Countertop basins can be mounted on a shelf or 'table', offering a similar option, but if mounted on a cupboard, then the person will not be as close and will have to lean to reach the bowl and taps.

The height of the wall-hung basin or countertop is more flexible than those mounted on pedestals. There are height-adjustable (rise-and-fall) basins; manual, gas-assisted and powered lift options provide flexibility to meet need and any price constraints. Ideally the user will be able to operate the mechanism themselves, and designs are available with remote controls as well as fixed operating points.

The design and shape of the basin affect use. For countertop designs the height of the basin varies; for a person with restricted shoulder range of movement or limited upper limb function, a shallower design will be more suitable. This type of design is probably not suitable for someone who rests their forearms on the basin as the rim of the bowl is narrow and will be uncomfortable as pressure is not spread evenly.

Standard basin designs may offer similar issues but there are options with shallower bowls and wider sides that provide support for forearms. There are specialist accessible designs, but ergonomic designs are becoming more mainstream, providing more choice, and they are aesthetically less 'clinical'.

Taps are discussed in more detail later in this chapter, but options for emptying the basin after use do need to be discussed. The 'traditional' plug and chain are now less common, with pop up or pull up wastes standard provision. The humble plug and chain have their place – easier for many if they do not have the reach, power or range of movement to operate other options. The chain is quite forgiving if the person lacks fine motor control or has a tremor, and they require less effort, although they may be more of a challenge to insert into the waste prior to filling the bowl. Pull lever/pull up wastes are often situated just in front of or behind the taps – awkward for most people to use, never mind those with a tremor or arthritic hands.

If you have a pop up waste in the basin in your home (or somewhere where people won't be wondering why you are taking quite so long to wash your hands!) stop and assess what is needed to operate it. Think about how this would impact on someone with reduced shoulder range of movement and/or with painful, arthritic finger joints.

The position of a basin in the bathroom is often between the tap end of the bath and the toilet. For people with limited knee and hip flexion, and who transfer into the bath in a seated position, basins with pedestals or half-pedestals can make transfers a challenge. A wall-hung basin may reduce or even resolve this issue.

Baths

Standard baths are not all created equal: lengths and widths vary, as do the internal dimensions, shape, tap and waste position. All these can impact on a person's ability to use the bath and your ability to prescribe appropriate bath supports. Where the bath design prevents the safe use of a bath lift or bath support, an alternative 'standard' design may be all that is needed.

Freestanding baths make a statement in a bathroom but are often deeper, making independent transfers difficult, and requiring caregivers to offer more assistance and adopt positions that may cause injury. Corner baths may be 'old fashioned', but there are plenty out there, and they definitely present challenges when selecting equipment. 'P-' and 'L'-shaped baths provide more space for over-bath showers but again, may make the choice of equipment difficult. Tap and waste positions need to be considered as well – if they are placed halfway along the side of the bath, use of equipment such as bath lifts and bath supports may be prevented. A basic rule of thumb is that a simple design works best: straight sides, an end that is not too steep an angle, the internal base of the bath as wide as possible, and taps and waste situated at one end of the bath.

Specialist baths including walk-in designs are often promoted as a 'simple and effective' option to replace the standard bath. A door in the side panel means that there is no requirement to step over to access the bath. The disadvantage of this design is that to use the door the bath has to be empty, so users have to sit and wait for the bath to fill...and then to empty. This increases the chance of someone's body temperature dropping, as well as significantly extending the length of time bathing takes. Generally, these baths are not practical, and in our experience, rarely recommended.

> Never say never! For the first time in 20+ years working in housing I suggested a team member consider recommending this type of bath. The reason for this was to meet the needs of different family members with one adaptation. One family member was unable to transfer in and out of the bath and required assistance, even with a bath lift. They preferred a shower as they could then be fully independent. The second family member had an arthritic condition that was eased by a warm bath, and they could transfer in and out independently. The walk-in bath resolved the need to achieve this within a limited space.

Standard bath designs require caregivers to kneel, stoop, bend and reach when they are assisting someone to bathe, which is not ideal, as it can result in musculoskeletal injury. A plinth raising the bath to a suitable working height may resolve this, but then may only suit the needs of some caregivers depending on their height and build. Additionally, raising the bath will increase the difficulty of transferring in and out for all users. Height-adjustable baths partially resolve this issue. They are designed with similar dimensions to standard baths, but rise to a suitable working height for caregivers. These baths come with a selection of accessories such as shower mixers, integral bath seats or lifts, internal platforms and integral changing or shower benches.

Bath lifts are items of equipment, and, as noted, the shape of the bath impacts on the ability to prescribe them. Fixed bath-side hoists pose similar challenges (and may be considered by some as an adaptation rather than equipment). The support is situated adjacent to the side of the bath and then the seat is raised over the bath, with the person in situ. If the shape of the bath or the incline at one end is too steep, the lift may have to be situated halfway down the bath, reducing the space to sit, which makes it an uncomfortable experience.

Taps

Baths and basins require water, and that requires taps. As with everything, design affects their usability. Options include two individual taps, each providing either hot or cold water. Mono mixer designs combine the two water supplies, with the person regulating the temperature by altering their flow. Individual taps mean that the hot water will flow at the temperature set at its source (either from a boiler or hot water tank). Mixer taps reduce risk, but it is always worth checking the water's temperature setting. Thermostatic taps limit the maximum temperature and may be appropriate where there is either a need to manage a skin condition or a risk of scalding or a burn.

Cross-head tap designs provide a secure grip but require rotational movement, which may be contraindicated for those with arthritic conditions in their hands and wrists. Lever taps can be operated in the vertical plane, but some designs may require a rotational movement. The ability to initiate this through pushing with a flat hand, forearm or other body part places less strain on hand and wrist joints.

Where there is an inability to reach the taps or to operate them, there is a range of sensor taps on the market. The sensors are usually sited on the front face of the tap, but there are designs with the sensor at the top of the tap – although issues with range of movement and reach would need consideration if this design was selected. Freestanding taps may offer a solution where reach is limited, as they do not have to be sited in the 'traditional' location at the rear of the basin.

And finally, push-type taps (timed valve) or foot-operated taps can be a solution. They are more usually found in public buildings, but if there are concerns about taps being left running, flooding, repetitive behaviour (see Chapter 17) or the ability to operate a cross-head or lever tap, these might be the answer you are looking for, as long as the person has the ability to depress the mechanism.

Showers

It can be easy to think that a level-access shower is the answer if someone has difficulty with bath transfers. This may well be the case, but do not discount the over-bath shower. Your observation and assessment will indicate if the person has the ability to bathe in this way. It is likely that equipment and grab rails (see Chapter 18) will be part of the solution to support safe transfers and independent bathing. Over-bath showers may be from a shower mixer tap on the bath, direct from the water supply or electric. Needless to say (but worth repeating), they must be thermostatically controlled. The choice of shower type will depend on a number of factors, such as the plumbing, power supply and the extent of work required to install them.

What is the difference between a level-access shower and a wet room? A level-access shower is a defined step-free shower area in a bathroom where the water must be limited within this area, although the flooring will usually extend throughout the room. A wet room is a room that is fully waterproof, which may or may not be step free. When discussing showering with those you are working with, ensure that they understand what is being recommended, as the mental image of a wet room is not necessarily the same as a level-access shower.

Shower heads, like everything these days, vary; there may be a single spray shower head or drench (rainfall) or both. A dual outlet system offers flexibility, but for any spray head there needs to be a long riser bar and extended shower hose to allow for use in both a seated and standing position. Drench shower heads are popular, and if the person is standing directly under them, they provide good coverage (with a decent-size shower head). Where they are less effective is if the bath design or equipment prevents the person sitting or standing directly below them. In this instance a shower head on a riser bar may be more appropriate, as the fall of the water is towards the person.

How the water is retained within a shower area is either via a curtain or screen. Shower curtains have their place as they can be moved out of the way to increase transfer space. Level-access showers will need a longer than standard curtain to minimize the spread of water. While people often prefer the appearance of shower screens, fixed panels on baths limit transfer options, and half-height shower screens may mean caregivers have to adopt awkward positions to provide assistance.

Equipment

There is a wide range of equipment that can be prescribed for use in the bathroom, but as there isn't the space here for a comprehensive list, we highlight two examples:

- Wall-hung changing or shower benches can be installed over baths, within shower areas or in 'dry' areas. The key aspects to consider are that the wall construction is appropriate (or is strengthened), what transfer and workspace is available when the bench is lowered, and ensuring that lighting is not directly in the person's eyes when they are reclined.

- For those who are unable to dry themselves independently, wall or ceiling air dryers can be installed. If the person can change their position to benefit from the warm air flow, they are effective. If a person still requires assistance from a caregiver to dry after a bath or shower, we would advise that this is over-provision.

Heating and ventilation

Effective heating is essential in a bathroom. This is a room where we wear few or no clothes (perhaps stating the obvious?), and the impact of stepping out of water and evaporation increases the rapidity of temperature change. Heating is usually via a radiator or a plumbed in or electric towel rail. It is also possible to install under-floor heating. The key considerations are the person's ability to control the temperature level and when the room is heated. There is little point in having heating if it is not warming the room during periods of use. Review the position of heat sources, as prolonged direct touch may cause burns, which is possibly an issue if the radiator is close to the toilet. Additionally, if a radiator or towel rail is close to a transfer point, they may be inappropriately used as a support.

And a final note on ventilation. Damp, musty bathrooms are not ideal and are detrimental to health, so enabling the room to be ventilated is essential. Windows are often awkward to reach, so there is a role for assistive technology and ensuring extractor fans are effective. However, extractor fans may run at a pitch that is uncomfortable for some.

This chapter has explored some of the barriers and enablers to access bathing. Facilitating bathing is a key area of practice for occupational therapists working in social care and housing. The impact of barriers to bathing can affect both physical and mental wellbeing, and a reliance on others alters the balance of a relationship. Don't forget the importance of bathing within cultural or belief systems. Ensuring that this room promotes personal care in a way that reflects the needs and wishes of the person has a significantly wider impact than simply the maintenance of personal cleanliness.

23

Bedroom Adaptations

Knowledge check

* Is there a minimum size specified for a bedroom?

* Can children over the age of 10 share a bedroom?

* Can a gas fire be installed in a room used for sleeping?

Although we spend a significant amount of time in our bedrooms (especially as teenagers), this chapter is surprisingly short, as most needs can be met with equipment.

Sharing a bedroom

There appears to be an expectation that children will have their own space rather than sharing a bedroom. The NSPCC (2022) recommends that children of the opposite sex over the age of 10 should not share bedrooms, although this is not, as yet, stated in any legislation. In social housing the picture is clearer (although it differs between the home nations), with limits on who can and cannot share rooms according to age and gender.

Parents often share a bedroom with their new-born baby, and this may continue when the child is a toddler. Generally, we would not expect any child older than this to be sharing a bedroom with parents, as there is an expectation that all will be entitled to space and privacy. However, where a child or young person has complex needs, the boundary of age-appropriate sharing can become blurred. Parents may consider the level of oversight and intervention required outweighs the impact on privacy and dignity. We, on the other hand, worry about restrictive practice.

You should be able to resolve this, although the discussion will need to be handled sensitively. It may be that equipment to support turning in bed removes the need to address comfort. If you find that the need to share arises from anxiety around a need to respond to a child's need, this may be resolved via assistive technology, an intercom or mobile phone. These are still restrictive if they are constantly monitored, but dependent on the child's ability it may be that the system is only used when parents feel they need support.

If a speedy response to a medical emergency is the concern, installing a door between two bedrooms may provide the answer. Ideally this would remain closed overnight, but accept that in many cases this will remain open. The pragmatist will say that there is now a choice for the door to be closed, which is an improvement on the parent sleeping in the same room. Not ideal, but an improvement nonetheless.

Space and dividing rooms

A request may be made to divide up a 'large' bedroom to provide an additional bedroom. At first sight this can appear a sensible (and cost-effective) option, but there are a few things to consider:

- The location of the dividing wall.

- The location of the new door.

- The location of lighting and electrical points.

- Natural light – is a second window in the 'right' place?

- Size of the resulting rooms.

A technical specification for room sizes in new-build properties has been published (HM Government 2022). While this is advisory and local authorities may apply a higher standard, it gives a guide as to what you should aim to achieve. There is no specific room size for younger children, but the minimum for a person over 10 years old is 6.51m², bearing in mind you should be seeking to meet long-term need.

Safety

Requests for additional bedrooms often result from safety concerns where a person exhibits behaviours that challenge as they will be unsupervised overnight, which may place younger or vulnerable siblings at risk. This could be linked with recommendations to ensure that the bedroom environment is safe (see Chapter 17).

Gas fires

A decision to sleep on the ground floor is often a pragmatic and sensible choice; however, where there is a gas fire, this needs to meet regulations introduced in 1998 (HSE 2022). Many landlords will require the gas appliance to be decommissioned as a matter of course if a room is utilized for sleep.

Through floor lifts

Through floor lifts enable many to access the first (or higher) floors in a property. Aside from the practicality of space on the ground floor and in the room it travels up to, also consider the noise level when this is in use. If used when others in the household are asleep, they may find this disturbs them.

If you consider that we sleep an average of six hours per night, some more, some less, this is a short chapter given that this is a quarter of the 24-hour day. The reason for this is that we have provided answers to many of the adaptations within other chapters of the book, so have tried to avoid repeating ourselves.

24

Case Scenarios

These case studies are written for you to use in conjunction with the set of architectural drawings (see Figures 27 and 28), to practise your evaluation of an environment from drawings. Remember that sometimes referrals identify an issue, but your knowledge and experience indicate that there are other aspects to consider and address.

We have not provided any 'correct' answers. You will be bringing your knowledge and experience, just as you would for casework. If you are unsure what the next steps should be, this is an opportunity to discuss this with a colleague or in supervision – all good CPD.

We accept that these are very concise summaries, so you may want to flesh out the narrative or perhaps use a situation from your current casework.

The architectural drawings (Figures 27 and 28) are reproduced online and available at https://library.jkp.com/redeem, using the code EDKQQWA.

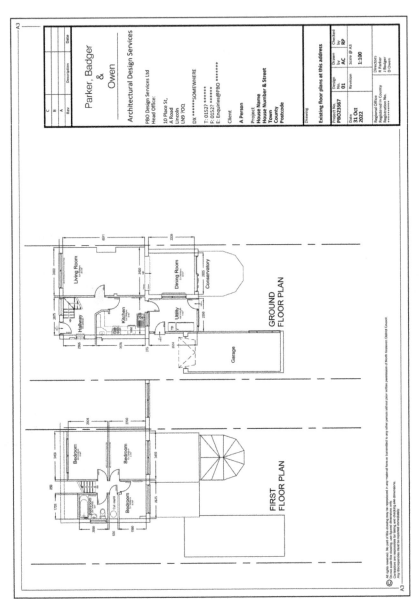

FIGURE 27. GROUND AND FIRST FLOOR PLAN VIEW
Source: North Kesteven District Council/Andrea Cox

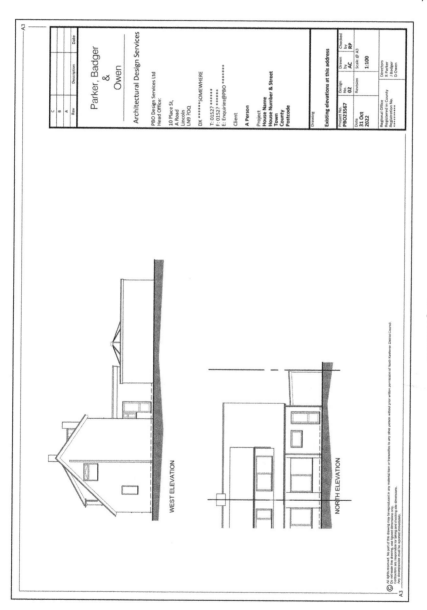

FIGURE 28. ELEVATION VIEW

Source: North Kesteven District Council/Andrea Cox

Have a read through, select a scenario, review the architectural drawings and then:

- Identify existing enablers.

- Note key barriers to occupations.

- Consider what you would include in your recommendation for adaptation.

Scenario 1

A is a child aged nine with diagnoses of muscular dystrophy and autism. He is still independently mobile but falls more frequently and has increasing levels of fatigue. He lives with his parents and younger brother aged five, who is undergoing tests to confirm if he has muscular dystrophy. The family has a cat and five goldfish. Both parents work full time.

Identified needs on occupational therapy referral

A referral was made following physiotherapist advice asking for general adaptations, but the parents were unsure as to what was needed.

Physical presentation

A is mobile with a wide gait, becoming unsteady with fatigue. His mobility is affected by muscle spasms and cramps. He is able to complete transfers independently, although is finding rising from sitting more difficult, especially if he has been playing at floor level.

Cognition and understanding

A has no cognitive impairment, and his verbal communication and comprehension are appropriate for his age.

Social-emotional aspects

A is aware that his abilities are changing, and will not discuss this outside of his family. He turns away if a professional asks him any questions. He is anxious that he has 'passed' his condition on to his brother.

Meaningful roles and occupations

A attends mainstream school but finds the school day tiring. In his free time he enjoys being part of a Cub Scouts group, swimming and Minecraft.

Activities of daily living

A does not need physical assistance with personal care activities. He can prepare snacks and drinks. A's parents are keen that he take on roles and responsibilities to earn pocket money. Currently he is expected to make his bed, tidy his room and feed the goldfish.

Parent/partner/caregiver aspects

A's parents would like him to have a similar childhood to his peers, so want to limit the level of adaptations in the home at this time; however, they would like a plan in place so that when adaptations are required, they can be completed quickly.

Identified outcomes

- Identify future adaptations to support A when he is a full-time wheelchair user.

- Promote A's continued independence in personal care.

- Maintain a 'typical' house rather than medicalize the home environment.

Scenario 2

B is a 16-year-old girl with a diagnosis of spastic quadriplegia. B attends a special school and plans to attend the local university to study English Literature. She is a member of the local Boccia club, and enjoys pamper sessions with her mother. B lives with her parents, pet cat and dog.

Identified needs on occupational therapy referral

B requires access to her bedroom and the family bathroom.

Physical presentation

B is tall and has a slim build. She is unable to independently mobilize or weight bear, and has to be carried upstairs. She is hoisted in and out of the bath. Indoors she is moved between rooms in a seating system or wheelchair; outdoors she uses a powered wheelchair.

Cognition and understanding

B can indicate her needs through vocalizations and facial expressions, and has strong opinions on how her care needs should be met. At school she uses eye-gaze technology, but prefers not to use this at home.

Social-emotional aspects

B has a positive outlook but becomes anxious when discussing change. She wants to be more independent and have control over some aspects of life, but recognizes that she will continue to need a high level of caregiver support.

Meaningful roles and occupations

At home B likes to spend time watching television, listening to audiobooks and pamper sessions with her mother. She also enjoys going out to the shops and meeting up with friends.

Activities of daily living

B requires full support from her parents with all activities of daily living.

Parent/partner/caregiver aspects

B's parents recognize that she should have more choice and control in her life, and that they can no longer complete manual transfers.

Identified outcomes

- Safe transfers for B between the ground and first floor.

- Increased mobility for B within the ground floor.

- B to have independent access to the community.

Scenario 3

C is 13 years old presenting with behaviours that challenge. He has diagnoses of tuberous sclerosis and learning disabilities. Following seizures he is sleepy and not mobile, and after periods of high seizure activity he regresses, losing some abilities that need to be relearned. C lives with his mother, stepfather and twin sisters aged 18 months.

Identified needs on occupational therapy referral

C requires assistance with personal care and transfers after seizures.

Physical presentation

C is mobile with an unsteady gait, but after seizures he is non-weight-bearing.

Cognition and understanding

C does not understand his changing abilities, becoming frustrated when he requires additional support.

Social-emotional aspects

When C's routine is altered he becomes anxious and demonstrates self-injurious behaviours (head-banging on radiators) and aggression towards others.

Meaningful roles and occupations

C prefers a set routine at home where he can watch his favourite television shows in a room on his own. He does not like to spend time outdoors.

Activities of daily living

C usually requires verbal prompts to manage personal care tasks and toileting. After a seizure he is incontinent and fully reliant on caregivers during the recovery period.

Parent/partner/caregiver aspects

C's parents are concerned that he is losing skills and independence, and are worried about the safety of his siblings.

Identified outcomes

- Access to bathing for C following seizures.

- Transfers for C following seizures.

- Minimizing the impact of C's anxiety.

Scenario 4

D is 22 years old and paraplegic (T11) following a vehicle collision two years ago. D is planning to return to the local university to complete her science degree. She had been living in student accommodation during term time, but has decided to remain in the family home in the long term. D lives with her parents, brother (18) and sister (13), utilizing the dining room and conservatory as her living space.

Identified needs on occupational therapy referral

To maximize independence for D throughout the home, but especially her access to toileting and bathing.

Physical presentation

D is non-weight-bearing and is able to transfer independently through sliding transfers. She mobilizes in a manual wheelchair. D has no control over her bowel and bladder functions; she is independent in managing her catheter, bowel evacuation and personal hygiene.

Cognition and understanding

D's injury did not affect her cognitive abilities. She understands that she will remain a wheelchair user and the importance of maintaining skin integrity and managing bladder and bowel health.

Social-emotional aspects

D is outgoing and has a positive outlook on life. She continues to access counselling services and has linked with spinal injury charities for support.

Meaningful roles and occupations

D wishes to complete her science degree. She has a wide circle of friends who visit and take her out socializing and to the cinema. Previously she enjoyed baking and making cocktails.

Activities of daily living

Currently D is limited by lack of access to the bathroom and her personal care is managed by strip washing and a commode. She uses her grandmother's level-access shower three times a week when her parents are available to drive her there. She cannot prepare meals at home.

Parent/partner/caregiver aspects

D's parents are fully supportive of her wish to be independent in the family home.

Identified outcomes

- D to have independent access in and out of the home.
- Access for D to bathing and toileting facilities.
- The ability for D to prepare meals and drinks.

Scenario 5

E is 35 years old with a diagnosis of relapsing remitting multiple sclerosis. He continues to work in his IT role, but has recently reduced his working hours and is supported to work from home. He drives an unadapted car. E is a keen football supporter and with his partner enjoys pub quizzes, visiting the cinema and meals out with friends. E lives with his partner who is expecting their first child. She works full-time as a hairdresser, but expects to reduce her hours after maternity leave. They live close to both sets of parents who have offered childcare support in the future.

Identified needs on occupational therapy referral

E requires wheelchair access to and within the home.

Physical presentation

E's symptoms vary but include fatigue, visual disturbance, altered/reduced sensation, tremor (left hand), muscle spasms and stiffness, cognitive changes and low mood. His unsteady gait means that he is increasingly using a wheelchair outdoors, but 'furniture walks' in his home. He is experiencing difficulty in climbing stairs when fatigued.

Cognition and understanding

E understands the impact and implications of his diagnosis. There are times when his episodic memory and speed of information processing are impaired.

Social-emotional aspects

E wishes to retain his current lifestyle, as his social circle and activities are important. He has periods of low mood and irritability, and has not sought support for this as yet. He is concerned he will become 'a burden' on his partner.

Meaningful roles and occupations

It is important to E that he plays an active part in caring for their child once it is born. He intends to continue in his current employment as he feels they are supportive.

Activities of daily living

Currently E is fully independent in all activities of daily living, but as he is left hand dominant, the tremor is a concern.

Parent/partner/caregiver aspects

E's partner is supportive of his wish to remain independent and continue working. She is concerned that this will lead to increased fatigue, and that this may impact on their family life once their child is born.

Identified outcomes

- Maintain E's independence in personal care.

- Prepare E for increased use of a wheelchair.

- Enable an active childcare role for E.

Scenario 6

F is 40 years old and has a diagnosis of retinitis pigmentosa. She lives alone following a recent divorce. Her field of vision has reduced significantly and she now has central (tunnel) vision, poor night vision and light sensitivity to bright lights. Following her divorce, F has realized the level of reliance she had on her partner, and wishes to become more independent.

Identified needs on occupational therapy referral

F requires independence in all aspects of daily life.

Physical presentation

F has full mobility and range of movement; however, she has had a recent fall, which has affected her confidence.

Cognition and understanding

F has no cognitive impairment and understands the implications of her diagnosis.

Social-emotional aspects

Following F's divorce she is increasingly socially isolated and has a high level of anxiety in managing the daily tasks her partner used to complete. Her anxiety is also related to concerns about personal safety, now she lives alone.

Meaningful roles and occupations

F enjoyed her role in maintaining the home, but recognizes that she now needs to learn new skills. She enjoys listening to Radio 4 and audiobooks.

She spends time on forums relating to her diagnosis, and has a circle of friends resulting from this.

Activities of daily living
F is independent in housework tasks, as this was the area of household management she has always managed; her ex-partner took responsibility for shopping, cooking and the garden.

Parent/partner/caregiver aspects
F does not have family in the area and her ex-partner has moved away.

Identified outcomes

- Home safety for F.

- Kitchen activities for F.

- Bathroom adaptation to reduce the impact of glare for F.

Scenario 7
G is 59 years old and obese, weighing over 190kg (30 stone). He has recently left his job due to his health conditions. He lives with his 62-year-old partner who works part-time as a hotel receptionist.

Identified needs on occupational therapy referral
G requires access to bathing.

Physical presentation
G has an 'apple' body shape with a significant girth. He has osteoarthritis in his spine, shoulder, hips and knees. He is short of breath on exertion (mobilizing and transfers). He has a wide gait and has fallen recently and been unable to rise independently. He has a bowel condition, which results in urgency and frequency, with loose stools.

Cognition and understanding
G has some difficulty in recalling and retaining information. His wife believes this may be due to dementia, but G will not discuss this with his GP, saying it is part of the adjustment to his retirement.

Social-emotional aspects

G initially presents as cheerful and positive, but in conversation becomes tearful about his current situation. His previous social life was linked to his job role, and their family live some distance away. He is reluctant to discuss the impact of his weight and arthritic conditions.

Meaningful roles and occupations

G spends his days watching sport on the television. He had never taken an active role in managing the household, and does not think he is physically able to contribute now.

Activities of daily living

G says that he is independent, but his wife advises that he does need assistance after a bowel movement, as he doesn't always get upstairs in time. Also, she advises that he strip washes as he cannot rise from the base of the bath. He used to have an allotment, but gave that up due to his arthritis and shortness of breath.

Parent/partner/caregiver aspects

G's wife is concerned that with lack of activity G's weight will increase, and without meaningful activity he will become depressed. She would like him to be active in managing the household tasks.

Identified outcomes

- G to have access to toileting.

- G to have access to bathing.

- Access to the first floor for G.

Scenario 8

H is 82 and with a diagnosis of Alzheimer's disease and has limited sight and hearing, chronic obstructive pulmonary disease (COPD) and is frail. She lives with her husband (93) who has a heart condition, and a daughter (55), who works night shifts.

Identified needs on occupational therapy referral

General advice on home safety is needed as H wanders and will attempt to prepare meals. H also needs a stairlift to access the first floor.

Physical presentation

H is petite in stature and has lost weight recently due to poor appetite. She is mobile with a walking stick, but frequently 'furniture walks' as she cannot always locate her stick. She is able to manage the stairs with assistance, but becomes short of breath.

Cognition and understanding

H is unable to retain new information and has difficulty in recall of names. She does not recognize herself in the mirror and mistakes her husband for his father. She does not have insight into her condition.

Social-emotional aspects

H becomes anxious and distressed when left alone. She does not recognize the passage of time and will often demand a meal soon after eating. When this is explained to her, she accuses her husband and daughter of cruelty. When people visit the home, she will tell them that she is being abused and kept prisoner. She will not consider time outside of the home or carer support.

Meaningful roles and occupations

H spends her time listening to programmes on the television. She is spending increasing amounts of time asleep in bed.

Activities of daily living

H is able to manage bathing and toileting independently, although her family are concerned she will fall when in the bathroom. She is able to dress and undress herself, but cannot choose clothes to wear as she becomes anxious over decision-making. Her meals and drinks are prepared for her.

Parent/partner/caregiver aspects

H's husband is concerned about her safety when he goes out during the day; however, he feels the time outside of the house is important for his own wellbeing. As his daughter is asleep during the day, he is worried that his wife's need for reassurance will affect his daughter's sleep pattern, which could affect the daughter's ability to work.

Identified outcomes

- Kitchen safety for H.

- Bathroom safety for H.

- Access to the first floor for H.

Concluding Thoughts

Reflecting on the information collated within this book, we must admit that even though we wrote the proposal for this book, we are surprised at the wide range of topics and information that have relevance for housing adaptations.

We have not positioned ourselves as 'experts' in the field of adaptations; more that we have recognized that the transition into this area of occupational therapy practice can be challenging, especially as some practitioners work in small, isolated teams, lacking the benefits of close working relationships with more experienced colleagues.

As reflective practitioners we had considered our previous experience and acquired knowledge, and recognized that writing this book would provide us with new learning opportunities. Some information built on existing knowledge, while the reading and research for topics outside of our everyday work remits introduced new knowledge. Even though there was no direct relevance to our day jobs, much of the information is transferable, informing and supporting the development of our practice. This is especially true of the chapters on professional reasoning, designing for a diverse population and sensitive conversations – topics that form part of our professional practice, but, due to the pressures of casework, are ones we rarely have time to stop and consider in depth.

This also applies to the start of our journey through the book, a reflection on the meaning of home. We recognize the positive impact of the changes we make, but contemplating the importance and meaning of the home environment to the person we are supporting is part of a holistic assessment and our person-centred practice.

The book is a collaborative effort, reflecting the multi-disciplinary and cross-profession working practices intrinsic to housing adaptations. Occupational therapists' ability to communicate and navigate complex situations enables the voice and preferences of those we support to be reflected in the resulting adaptations, and this has been the case with this book.

As we conclude, we must remember that every situation is unique, and that our role as occupational therapists is to take the available information, apply it to the person's circumstances and, through a process of review, discussion and revision, identify the most suitable solution.

Glossary

A

Accessibility: The ability for a person to enter or use a space or facility.

Activity (or task) analysis: Observation of an activity that is then broken down into its component parts, enabling understanding of the abilities needed to successfully complete it.

Adaptation: Physical alteration or addition to a building to promote accessibility.

Architectural drawing: A drawing or schematic depicting a building; often referred to by the generic term 'plan'.

Assessment: The process of observation of a person, discussion of their needs and abilities and following this, completion of a written report.

B

Barrier: An aspect of the home environment that prevents a person gaining access or completing an activity.

C

Caregiver: A person providing support to an individual who is unable to complete an activity independently.

Co-production: The process of service providers working with an individual to facilitate an outcome.

D

Disability: A physical or mental impairment that has a 'substantial' and 'long-term' negative effect on a person's health, wellbeing and their ability to complete everyday tasks.

Disabled Facilities Grant (DFG): Funding for adaptations to privately owned or housing association properties; mandated under the Housing Grants, Construction and Regeneration Act 1996 in England, Wales and Northern Ireland.

Disabled Facilities Grant (DFG) recommendation: Typically completed by an occupational therapist working in social care outlining the assessed needs to be addressed by an adaptation. This forms the basis for the adaptation scheme proposed to address identified needs.

E

Equipment: Aids and equipment specifically designed to promote independence and minimize the impact of a person's disability.

Enabler: An adaptation, advice or item of equipment that reduces the impact of barriers (see above), allowing a person to complete desired activities.

Environmental assessment: An assessment of a property to evaluate the enablers and barriers in regard to an individual's assessed needs. Typically used when a person is seeking rehousing by a social housing provider.

Evidence-based practice: The process by which decisions are made based on information that is current, relevant and valid.

F

Fused spur: A switch that isolates electrical equipment from a mains supply. Examples of use include powered equipment in a bath or shower room, and for installation of some tracked hoists.

H

Holistic assessment: An assessment that considers all aspects of a person's situation – physical, social and emotional.

Homeowner: A person who owns their property; also known as an owner-occupier.

Housing provider: Social housing provider, also known as a registered social housing provider or housing association.

I

Inclusive Design: An approach that designs for the widest range of people considering age, ability and situation; also known as Universal Design.

M

Medical model of disability: An approach that focuses on the impact of an individual's disability or medical condition as the creator of the barriers the individual faces.

Models of practice: The theoretical applications underpinning occupational therapy practice.

O

Occupation(s): The activities an individual needs or wants to complete.

Objectives: The outcomes that have been identified following an assessment of needs and agreed with the individual being supported.

P

Part M of the Building Regulations: Approved Document M – Access to and use of buildings: Volume 1 – Dwellings Regulations applied during the build process that influence the accessibility of the property.

Person-Environment-Occupation-Performance (PEOP) model: An occupational therapy model of practice focusing on occupational performance.

Professional reasoning: The thought processes employed to understand what is being observed, and to determine the next steps to be taken.

Property: A domestic dwelling that may be owner-occupied or rented.

R

Royal College of Occupational Therapists (RCOT): The professional body for occupational therapists.

Recommendation for adaptation: Submitted following an assessment of need; this outlines the barriers a person is experiencing and the areas of a property that require adaptation to address these.

Regulatory reform order (RRO): Legislation enabling the provision of discretionary grants either to 'top up' a Disabled Facilities Grant (DFG), to remove the need for means tests for some adaptations or to provide flexibility for adaptations that may not sit within the DFG criteria in England and Wales.

Rehousing: The process by which someone is allocated a property, which either matches their identified needs or has the ability to be adapted to achieve this.

Restrictive practice: An action, recommendation, adaptation or equipment that limits an individual's ability to make a choice. The Mental Capacity Act 2005 guides occupational therapists to consider this in relation to the person's chronological age, not their diagnosis or ability. In the context of adaptations this includes stable doors and locks.

S

Scale: The measurement used to depict an accurate representation of a structure at a practical size, enabling an understanding of the space available.

Scale drawing: A drawing utilizing a specific scale, providing an accurate representation of the space.

Sketch drawing: A freehand drawing depicting a room or floor plan.

Social housing: Rental properties provided by a local authority or housing association where the rental rates reflect the needs of the local population, with an aim to be affordable.

Social model of disability: An approach that considers disabilities to be caused by environmental and societal barriers.

Stairlift: A tracked mechanism installed on a staircase to enable a person to ascend and descend in a seated position.

T

Tenant: A person who rents their home from a landlord.

Tenure: The conditions by which a property is occupied; for domestic dwellings this is either owner-occupied or rented.

Theoretical framework: These conceptualize the models and schools of thought that underpin the practice of occupational therapy.

Through floor lift: In domestic dwellings these are generally not enclosed with a shaft transitioning between floors, allowing for use in a standing or seated position or in a wheelchair.

Tracked hoist: Hoist units installed on a track allowing for pick up or lowering positions to be in different locations. Types include ceiling track, wall-hung or gantry, and may consist of a single track or H frame/XY systems, which provide greater flexibility.

Transfers: The movement of a person from one item of equipment to another. These may be independent, where the person does not require assistance, manually assisted by a carer or supported via equipment such as a hoist and sling or a standing aid.

U

Usability: Design of equipment or an environment that focuses on the aspects that ensure that those interacting with it can do so with minimum effort (physical and cognitive). The five key aspects are highlighted as effectiveness, efficiency, engaging, tolerant of user error and being easy to learn.

Appendix: Occupational Therapy Assessments

★ Occupational therapy initial assessment

Section 1		
Person assessed (service user/patient/client)	Date of birth	Unique identifier (e.g., NHS no.)
Date and time of assessment	Assessor	Role
Location of the assessment	Home address	Others contributing to the assessment

Section 2
Reason for assessment

Has consent for the assessment been given?   Yes/No/N/A
Does the person understand the reason for the assessment?   Yes/No/N/A
If the answer is 'No' or 'N/A', explain the reasoning for continuing with the assessment:
Person's home and social situation

Medical history, diagnoses and disability

Height:	(cm)	Weight:	(kg)

Communication, comprehension and language (including vision and hearing)

Involved professionals/support services

Property information

Type of property:	Homeowner/tenant
Access: ramp/stairs/lift	No. of bedrooms

Adaptations/equipment previously provided

Person's self-reported areas of need and preferred outcomes

Section 3

Activities of daily living

Mobility (including stairs)	

What do they think may assist them in this area?

Transfers (including methods and hoisting)	

What do they think may assist them in this area?

Toileting (including continence)	

What do they think may assist them in this area?

Bathing/showering (including preferred method)	

What do they think may assist them in this area?

Personal care (including dental and hair care)	

What do they think may assist them in this area?

Sleep (including type of bed)	

What do they think may assist them in this area?

Meals and nutrition (including ability to swallow)	

What do they think may assist them in this area?

Work/education/leisure	

What do they think may assist them in this area?

Other relevant information	

Section 4

Identified areas of need

1.
2.
3.
...

Agreed objectives

1.
2.
3.
...

Analysis and professional reasoning

Section 5

Date of report	Date shared with person

Report completed by	Signed

★ Occupational therapy environmental assessment

Section 1		
Person (service user/ patient/client)	Date of birth	Unique identifier (e.g., NHS no.)

Date of assessment	Assessor		Role

Location of the assessment	Others present	Role and contact details

Section 2
Reason for environmental assessment (including if rehousing/property purchase/ property exchange and who requested the assessment)

Tenure/housing provider's contact details

Type of property

House: Terraced/semi-detached/detached/townhouse

Bungalow: Single-storey/dormer

Flat/apartment: State floor: Maisonette/bedsit/studio/high-rise

Stairs/lift

Other:

Outcome of environmental assessment

Is this property suitable for the named person?	Yes/No
Does it require adaptations to meet assessed need?	Yes/No

If yes, please state what adaptations have been identified:

If discussed with the housing provider/housing provider's representative during the assessment visit, have the above recommendations been agreed in principle?

Discussed and agreed with:

If the property is not suitable, provide reasoning here:

Area of the property/room	Image(s) (insert as required)
Approach	Driveway/path/surface finishes

Main entrance	Advise if other than front door/steps/ramp/rails/porch etc.

Entrance hall	Location of stairs/width of hallway etc.

Family room	

Dining room	Is this suitable for use as a room for sleeping?

Kitchen	

Utility	

Stairs/access to first or other floors	Second stair rail/stairlift/through floor lift

Bedroom 1	

Bedroom 2	

Add sections for additional bedrooms

Bathroom	Type of bath/shower, en suite/family bathroom

Toilet (if separate to bathroom)	Ground floor/first floor/en suite

Rear access	Steps/ramp/rails

Outside space	Garden/yard/private/communal/access

Heating	Gas/storage heaters/back boiler/ground or air source heat pump

Other	

Section 4	
Date of environmental assessment report	Date(s) shared with person/housing provider

Report completed by	Signed

★ Occupational therapy risk evaluation

Section 1		
Person (service user/ patient/client)	Date of birth	Unique identifier (e.g., NHS no.)

Date of evaluation	Assessor	Role

Home address	Others contributing to the evaluation

Section 2
Reason(s) for risk evaluation

Has consent for the evaluation been given?   Yes/No/N/A

Does the person understand the reason for the evaluation?   Yes/No/N/A

If the answer is 'No' or 'N/A', explain the reasoning for continuing with the evaluation:

Person's home and social situation

Medical history, diagnoses and disability

Communication, comprehension and language (*including vision and hearing*)

Involved professionals/support services

Current situation

Area(s) of concern

Do concerns relate to:

Risk of injury ☐

Restrictive practice(s) ☐

Risk of injury and restrictive practice(s) ☐

Section 3

As practitioners, occupational therapists may become aware of activities and actions that have a risk of harm or injury to an individual. This evaluation assists in promoting independence by supporting positive risk taking while minimizing hazards.

Where an item of equipment, adaptation or practice is restrictive in nature, the Mental Capacity Act 2005 requires us to identify the least restrictive option that is appropriate to meeting the assessed needs of the person.

Mental Capacity Act 2005: www.legislation.gov.uk/ukpga/2005/9/contents

Capacity

- *Assume* capacity
- Identify if the person can *understand* the information
- Identify if the person can *retain* the information
- Can the person *use* the information to make a decision?
- Understand how and if the person can *communicate* their wishes

If a person has capacity, they can choose to make an unwise or risky decision.

Please outline how the person's (named above) capacity to make a decision has been supported:

Area of concern 1

Does this relate to risk of injury and/or restrictive practice(s) (*delete as appropriate*)

What is the impact of the behaviour or activity on them or on others? (*Include if identified risks are actual or potential*)

Identified solutions to minimize risk

1. Current arrangements

2. Option 2

3. Option 3

(*Additional rows to be added as required*)

Which is the least risky/least restrictive option?

Option:

Is it appropriate to continue with the current arrangements?
Is an alternative option recommended?

Provide your rationale:

Recommended option:

Occupational therapy actions to support this option

Other relevant information	

(*Additional rows to be added as required*)

Section 4	
Date of risk evaluation report	Date shared with person
Report completed by	Signed

References

Ainsworth, E. and de Jonge, D. (2011) *An Occupational Therapist's Guide to Home Modification Practice*. Thorofare, NJ: Slack Incorporated.

Atwal, S. (2022) 'World's tallest man, Sultan Kösen, celebrates 40th birthday.' Guinness World Records, 8 December. Available at www.guinnessworldrecords.com/news/2022/12/worlds-tallest-man-sultan-kosen-celebrates-40th-birthday-729062, accessed on 4 November 2022.

Baum, C.M., Christiansen, C.H. and Bass, J.D. (2015) 'The Person-Environment-Occupation-Performance (PEOP) Model.' In C.H. Christiansen, C.M. Baum and J.D. Bass (eds) *Occupational Therapy: Performance, Participation, and Well-Being* (4th edn, pp. 49–56). Thorofare, NJ: SLACK Incorporated.

Bougdah, H. and Salman, H.'A. (2018) *The Meaning of Home and Ways the Domestic Space Is Experienced*. ArchDesign 18, V International Architectural Design Conference, Istanbul: DAKAM (Eastern Mediterranean Academic Research Centre).

British Nutrition Foundation (2022) 'Dehydration in older people.' Available at www.nutrition. org.uk/life-stages/older-people/malnutrition-and-dehydration/dehydration-in-older-people, accessed on 12 December 2022.

BSI (British Standards Institute) (2018) 'BS 7671:2018 Requirements for Electrical Installations.' Available at www.bsigroup.com/en-GB/industries-and-sectors/construction-and-building/requirements-for-electrical-installations-iet-wiring-regulations, accessed on 12 December 2022.

BSI (2022) *Design for the Mind – Neurodiversity and the Built Environment – Guide*. Available at www.bsigroup.com/en-GB/standards/pas-6463/#:~:text=What%20does%20PAS%20 6463%3A2022,for%20independent%20or%20supported%20living, accessed on 29 November 2022.

Burrell, K. (2014) 'Spilling over from the street. Contextualizing domestic space in an inner-city neighborhood.' *Home Cultures 11*, 2, 145–166.

Buse, C., Balmer, A., Keady, J., Nettleton, S. and Swift, S. (2022) '"Ways of being" in the domestic garden for people living with dementia: Doing, sensing and playing.' *Ageing and Society.* doi: 10.1017/S0144686X22001489.

Campo, M., Fehlberg, B., Natalier, K. and Smyth, B. (2020) 'The meaning of home for children and young people after separation.' *Journal of Social Welfare and Family Law 42*, 3, 299–318.

Chalfont, G. and Walker, A. (2013) *Dementia Green Care Handbook of Therapeutic Design and Practice*. Sheffield: Safehouse Books.

Champagne, T. (2018) *Sensory Modulation in Dementia Care: Assessment and Activities for Sensory-Enriched Care*. London: Jessica Kingsley Publishers.

Chung, C., Chung, J., Dow, A., Wilson, J., *et al.* (2018) 'The introduction of cognitive screening when undertaking stairlift eligibility assessment.' *British Journal of Occupational Therapy 81*, 18.

Clutton, S., Grisbrooke, J. and Pengelly, S. (eds) (2006) *Occupational Therapy in Housing: Building on Firm Foundations*. New York: John Wiley & Sons.

Collins (2022) 'Common sense.' Available at www.collinsdictionary.com/dictionary/english/ common-sense, accessed on 4 December 2022.

Dalke, H. and Corso, A. (2013) *Making an Entrance: Colour, Contrast and the Design of Entrances to Homes of People with Sight Loss.* Kingston: Kingston University, London and Thomas Pocklington Trust. Available at www.pocklington-trust.org.uk/wp-content/ uploads/2020/10/Full-Making-an-Entrance.pdf, accessed on 1 January 2023.

Department for Communities (Northern Ireland) (2022) *Interdepartmental Housing Adaptations Design Toolkit.* Available at www.nihe.gov.uk/getattachment/b0653b86-7bd0-4dd8-b983-7c5215e4eca7/Housing-Adaptations-Design-Toolkit.pdf, accessed on 6 December 2022.

Department of Finance and Personnel (Northern Ireland) (2012) *Access to and Use of Buildings. Technical Booklet R. Building Regulations Guidance.* Available at www.buildingcontrol-ni.com/assets/pdf/TechnicalBookletR2012.pdf, accessed on 8 December 2022.

Després, C. (1991) 'The meaning of home: Literature review and directions for future research and theoretical development.' *Journal of Architectural and Planning Research 8*, 2, 96–115.

Dolenc, E. and Rotar-Pavlič, D. (2019) 'Frailty assessment scales for the elderly and their application in primary care: A systematic literature review'. *Slovenian Journal of Public Health 58*, 2, 91–100. doi: 10.2478/sjph-2019-0012.

Dovey, K. (1985) 'Home and Homelessness.' In I. Altman and C.M. Werner (eds) *Home Environments: Human Behavior and Environment*, Advances in Theory and Research, Volume 8 (pp.33–64). New York: Plenum Press.

Dow, A. (2020) 'Stairlift eligibility & #dementia: Overcoming an occupational therapist's dilemma.' Let's Talk about Dementia, 20 February. Available at https://letstalkaboutdementia.wordpress.com/2020/02/20/stairlift-eligibility-dementia-overcoming-an-occupational-therapists-dilemma, accessed on 1 January 2022.

DSDC (Dementia Services Development Centre) (2013) *Light and Lighting Design for People with Dementia* (3rd edn). Stirling: University of Stirling.

DSDC (2022) 'Environments for Ageing and Dementia Design Assessment Tool (EADDAT).' Available at www.dementia.stir.ac.uk/our-services/ea-ddat, accessed on 12 December 2022.

EHRC (Equality and Human Rights Commission) (2022) 'Housing and disabled people: Your rights.' Available at https://equalityhumanrights.com/en/advice-and-guidance/housing-and-disabled-people-your-rights, accessed on 24 December 2022.

Fänge, A. and Iwarsson, S. (2005) 'Changes in accessibility and usability in housing: An exploration of the housing adaptations process.' *Occupational Therapy International 12*, 1, 44–59.

Fox Mahoney, L. (2007) *Conceptualising Home: Theories, Laws and Policies.* London: Hart Publishing.

Fried, L.P., Tangen, C.M., Walston, J., Newman, A.B., Hirsch, C. and Gottdiener, J. (2001) 'Frailty in older adults: Evidence for a phenotype.' *The Journals of Gerontology. Series A, Biological Sciences and Medical Sciences 56*, 146–156.

Gallagher, A. (2013) 'Risk assessment: Enabler or barrier?' *British Journal of Occupational Therapy 76*, 7, 337–339.

Gallagher, J. (2022) 'Cold weather: What does an unheated room do to your body?' BBC News, 19 November. Available at www.bbc.co.uk/news/health-63602501, accessed on 6 December 2022.

Government Equalities Office (2013) *Disability: Equalities Act 2010 – Guidance on Matters to Be Taken into Account in Determining Questions Relating to the Definition of Disability.* Available at: www.gov.uk/government/publications/equality-act-guidance/disability-equality-act-2010-guidance-on-matters-to-be-taken-into-account-in-determining-questions-relating-to-the-definition-of-disability-html, accessed on 1 June 2023.

Greasley-Adams, C., Bowes, A., Dawson, A. and McCabe, L. (2014) *Good Practice in the Design of Homes and Living Spaces for People with Dementia and Sight Loss.* Thomas Pocklington Trust and University of Stirling. Available at www.pocklington-trust.org.uk/wp-content/ uploads/2020/10/Dementia-and-Sight-Loss-Design-Guide.pdf, accessed on 1 January 2023.

Gustafson, P. (2014) 'Place Attachment in an Age of Mobility.' In L.C. Manzo and L.P. Devine-Wright (eds) *Place Attachment: Advances in Theory, Methods and Applications* (pp.37–48). Abingdon: Routledge.

Hart, R.A. (1992) *Children's Participation: From Tokenism to Citizenship*. Innocenti Essay, No. 4. Florence: International Child Development Centre, UNICEF.

Henley, A. and Schott J. (1999) *Culture, Religion and Patient Care in a Multi-Ethnic Society: A Handbook for Professionals*. London: Age Concern Books.

Hindle, L. and Charlesworth, L. (2019) *UK Allied Health Professions Public Health Strategic Framework 2019–2024*. London: Allied Health Professions Federation. Available at www.ahpf.org.uk/files/UK%20AHP%20Public%20Health%20Strategic%20Framework%20 2019-2024.pdf, accessed on 3 April 2023.

HM Government (2016) *Access to and Use of Buildings. Approved Document M. The Building Regulations 2010*. Available at https://assets.publishing.service.gov.uk/government/uploads/ system/uploads/attachment_data/file/540330/BR_PDF_AD_M1_2015_with_2016_ amendments_V3.pdf, accessed on 3 December 2022.

HM Government (2022) 'Disabled Facilities Grant (DFG) delivery: Guidance for local authorities in England.' Available at www.gov.uk/government/publications/disabled-facilities-grant-dfg-delivery-guidance-for-local-authorities-in-england, accessed on 7 December 2022.

HSE (Health and Safety Executive) (1999) *Lifting Operations and Lifting Equipment Regulations (LOLER) 1998: Open Learning Guidance*. Available at www.hse.gov.uk/pubns/priced/loler. pdf, accessed on 1 December 2022.

HSE (2022) *Provision and Use of Work Equipment Regulations 1998 (PUWER)*. Available at www. hse.gov.uk/work-equipment-machinery/puwer.htm#:~:text=PUWER%20requires%20 that%20equipment%20provided,adequate%20information%2C%20instruction%20 and%20training, accessed on 1 December 2022.

Kelly, D.A. (2018) 'Impact of paved front gardens on current and future urban flooding.' *Journal of Flood Risk Management 11*, S434–S443.

Kitwood, T. and Brooker, D. (2019) *Dementia Reconsidered Revisited: The Person Still Comes First*. New York: McGraw-Hill Education.

Kylén, M., Löfqvist, C., Haak, M. and Iwarsson, S. (2019) 'Meaning of home and health dynamics among younger older people in Sweden.' *European Journal of Ageing 16*, 3, 305–315.

Levett-Jones, T., Hoffman, K., Dempsey, J., Jeong, S.Y.S., *et al.* (2010) 'The "five rights" of clinical reasoning: An educational model to enhance nursing students' ability to identify and manage clinically "at risk" patients.' *Nurse Education Today 30*, 6, 515–520.

Lim, Y.Z.G., Honey, A. and McGrath, M. (2022) 'The parenting occupations and purposes conceptual framework: A scoping review of "doing" parenting.' *Australian Occupational Therapy Journal 69*, 1, 98–111.

Maslin, S. (2021) *Designing Mind-Friendly Environments: Architecture and Design for Everyone*. London: Jessica Kingsley Publishers.

McDonald, S. (2022) 'Let's change how we talk about disability.' *OT News*, September, pp.24–27.

Met Office (2022) 'A milestone in UK climate history.' 22 July. Available at www.metoffice.gov.uk/ about-us/press-office/news/weather-and-climate/2022/july-heat-review#:~:text=This%20 was%20the%20first%20time,record%20of%2038.7%C2%B0C, accessed on 20 October 2022.

NHS (2022) 'Home adaptations.' Available at www.nhs.uk/conditions/social-care-and-support-guide/care-services-equipment-and-care-homes/home-adaptations, accessed on 1 December 2022.

NSPCC (2022) 'Sharing a bedroom: How to decide when it's okay for children to share a bedroom at home, away or on holiday and what you can do to help keep them safe.' Available at www.nspcc.org.uk/keeping-children-safe/in-the-home/sharing-a-bedroom, accessed on 10 December 2022.

ODPM (Office of the Deputy Prime Minister) (2003) CIR 05/2003 'Housing renewal.' Available at https://www.thenbs.com/PublicationIndex/documents/details?DocId=263969, accessed 5 September 2023.

Office for Health Improvement and Disparities (2022) 'Falls: Applying All Our Health.' Available at www.gov.uk/government/publications/falls-applying-all-our-health/falls-applying-all-our-health, accessed on 12 November 2022.

RCOT (Royal College of Occupational Therapists) (2016) *Care Act 2014: Guidance for Occupational Therapists – Disabled Facilities Grants.* Available at www.rcot.co.uk/practice-resources/rcot-publications/downloads/care-act-2014-dfg, accessed on 31 December 2022.

RCOT (2019) *Adaptations without Delay: A Guide to Planning and Delivering Home Adaptations Differently.* Available at www.rcot.co.uk/adaptations-without-delay, accessed on 1 January 2023.

RGA (Restricted Growth Association) (2022) 'About restricted growth.' Available at https://rgauk.org/about-restricted-growth, accessed on 14 October 2022.

Russell, R., Ormerod, M. and Newton, R. (2018) 'The development of a design and construction process protocol to support the home modification process delivered by occupational therapists.' *Journal of Aging Research.* doi: 10.1155/2018/4904379.

Schell, B.B. and Schell, J.W. (eds) (2008) *Clinical and Professional Reasoning in Occupational Therapy.* Philadelphia, PA: Lippincott Williams & Wilkins.

Scottish Government (2015) *Adaptations, Aids and Equipment.* Available at www.gov.scot/binaries/content/documents/govscot/publications/advice-and-guidance/2015/04/adaptations-aids-equipment-advice-note/documents/adaptations-aids-equipment-advice-note/adaptations-aids-equipment-advice-note/govscot%3Adocument/00476043.pdf, accessed on 1 January 2023.

Scottish Government (2021) 'Housing to 2040.' Available at www.gov.scot/publications/housing-2040-2, accessed on 1 January 2023.

Stark, S.L., Somerville, E., Keglovits, M., Smason, A. and Bigham, K. (2015) 'Clinical reasoning guideline for home modification interventions.' *American Journal of Occupational Therapy 69,* 2. doi: 10.5014/ajot.2015.014266.

UNICEF (1989) *The United Nations Convention on the Rights of the Child.* London: UNICEF UK.

Unsworth, C. and Baker, A. (2016) 'A systematic review of professional reasoning literature in occupational therapy.' *British Journal of Occupational Therapy 79,* 1, 5–16.

Veronese, N., Soysal, P., Stubbs, B., Marengoni, A., *et al.* (2018) 'Association between urinary incontinence and frailty: A systematic review and meta-analysis.' *European Geriatric Medicine 9,* 571–578.

Visser, R.C. (2019) 'Going beyond the dwelling: Challenging the meaning of home at the end of life.' *Anthropology and Aging 40,* 1, 5–10.

Wahl, H.W., Fänge, A., Oswald, F., Gitlin, L.N. and Iwarsson, S. (2009) 'The home environment and disability-related outcomes in aging individuals: What is the empirical evidence?' *The Gerontologist 49,* 3, 355–367.

Walker, M. (2022) 'Exploring how design can support the expression of personal aesthetic preferences in dementia.' *The Design Journal 25,* 5, 887–898.

Welsh Government (2019) *Housing Adaptations Service Standards.* Available at https://gov.wales/sites/default/files/publications/2019-04/housing-adaptations-standards-of-service.pdf, accessed on 13 March 2022.

Welsh Government (2022) *Physical Adaptation Grant Guidance for Registered Social Landlords.* Cardiff: Welsh Government.

Young, J. (2013) 'Frailty – what it means and how to keep well over winter months.' NHS England Blog, 20 December. Available at www.england.nhs.uk/blog/frailty/#:~:text=In%20medicine%2C%20frailty%20defines%20the,health%20and%20social%20care%20professionals, accessed on 16 November 2022.

Relevant legislation and guidance

Adaptations, Aids and Equipment: Advice Note (2015). Available at www.gov.scot/publications/adaptations-aids-equipment-advice-note, accessed on 9 May 2023.

Care Act 2014. Available at www.legislation.gov.uk/ukpga/2014/23/contents/enacted, accessed on 1 January 2023.

Children Act 1989. Available at www.legislation.gov.uk/ukpga/1989/41/contents, accessed on 9 May 2023.

Chronically Sick and Disabled Persons Act 1970. Available at www.legislation.gov.uk/ukpga/1970/44/contents, accessed on 1 January 2023.

Chronically Sick and Disabled Persons (Northern Ireland) Act 1978. Available at www.legislation.gov.uk/ukpga/1978/53, accessed on 1 January 2023.

Department for Communities (2016) *Adaptations Guide*. Available at www.communities-ni.gov.uk/adaptations-guide, accessed on 9 May 2023.

Disabled Persons (Northern Ireland) Act 1989. Available at www.legislation.gov.uk/ukpga/1989/10/contents, accessed on 1 January 2023.

Equality Act 2010. Available at www.legislation.gov.uk/ukpga/2010/15/contents, accessed on 1 January 2023.

Health and Personal Social Services (Northern Ireland) Order (1972). Available at www.legislation.gov.uk/nisi/1972/1265/contents, accessed on 15 December 2022.

Health and Safety at Work etc. Act 1974. Available at: www.legislation.gov.uk/ukpga/1974/37/contents, accessed on 9 May 2023.

Housing Grants, Construction and Regeneration Act 1996. Available at www.legislation.gov.uk/ukpga/1996/53/contents, accessed on 1 January 2023.

Housing (Scotland) Act 1987. Available at www.legislation.gov.uk/ukpga/1987/26/contents, accessed on 1 January 2023.

Housing (Scotland) Act 2001. Available at www.legislation.gov.uk/asp/2001/10/contents, accessed on 1 January 2023.

Housing (Scotland) Act 2006. Available at www.legislation.gov.uk/asp/2006/1/contents, accessed on 1 January 2023.

Human Rights Act 1998. Available at www.legislation.gov.uk/ukpga/1998/42/contents, accessed on 1 January 2023.

Mental Capacity Act 2005. Available at www.legislation.gov.uk/ukpga/2005/9/contents, accessed on 1 January 2023.

Public Bodies (Joint Working) (Scotland) Act 2014. Available at www.legislation.gov.uk/asp/2014/9/contents/enacted, accessed on 1 January 2023.

Social Services and Well-being (Wales) Act 2014. Available at www.legislation.gov.uk/anaw/2014/4/contents, accessed on 1 January 2023.

Technical Booklet R (2012). Available at www.finance-ni.gov.uk/sites/default/files/publications/dfp/Technical-booklet-R-Access-to-and-use-of-buildings-October-2012.pdf, accessed on 9 May 2023.

The Disabled Facilities Grants (Maximum Amounts and Additional Purposes) (England) Order 2008. Available at www.legislation.gov.uk/uksi/2008/1189/contents/made, accessed on 30 December 2022.

The Disabled Facilities Grants (Maximum Amounts and Additional Purposes) (Wales) Order 2008. Available at www.legislation.gov.uk/wsi/2008/2370/note/made, accessed on 9 May 2023.

The Health and Social Care Trusts (Establishment) (Amendment) Order (Northern Ireland) 2022. Available at www.legislation.gov.uk/nisr/2022/103/contents/made, accessed on 15 December 2022.

The Housing (Northern Ireland) Order (2003). Available at www.legislation.gov.uk/nisi/2003/412/contents, accessed on 15 December 2022.

The Manual Handling Operations Regulations 1992. Available at www.legislation.gov.uk/uksi/1992/2793/contents/made, accessed on 9 May 2023.

The Regulatory Reform (Housing Assistance) (England and Wales) Order 2002. Available at www.legislation.gov.uk/uksi/2002/1860/contents/made, accessed on 13 March 2022.

The Relevant Adjustments to Common Parts (Disabled Persons) (Scotland) 2020. Available at www.legislation.gov.uk/sdsi/2020/9780111043615/contents, accessed on 1 January 2023.

United Nations Convention on the Rights of Persons with Disabilities (2007). Available at https://social.desa.un.org/issues/disability/crpd/convention-on-the-rights-of-persons-with-disabilities-crpd, accessed on 1 June 2023.

Subject Index

Author Index